About the NCCN Guidelines for Patients®

NCCN National Comprehensive Cancer Network®

Did you know that top cancer centers across the United States work together to improve cancer care? This alliance of leading cancer centers is called the National Comprehensive Cancer Network® (NCCN®).

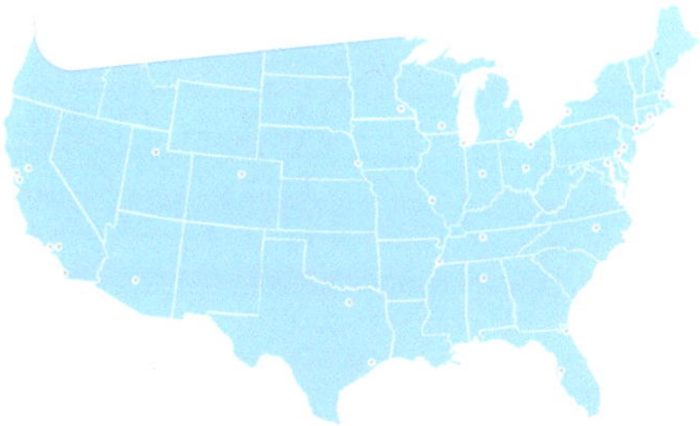

Cancer care is always changing. NCCN develops evidence-based cancer care recommendations used by health care providers worldwide. These frequently updated recommendations are the NCCN Clinical Practice Guidelines in Oncology (NCCN Guidelines®). The NCCN Guidelines for Patients plainly explain these expert recommendations for people with cancer and caregivers.

These NCCN Guidelines for Patients are based on the NCCN Clinical Practice Guidelines in Oncology (NCCN Guidelines®) for Central Nervous System Cancers, Version 1.2023 — March 24, 2023.

View the NCCN Guidelines for Patients free online
NCCN.org/patientguidelines

Find an NCCN Cancer Center near you
NCCN.org/cancercenters

Connect with us

Supporters

NATIONAL COMPREHENSIVE CANCER NETWORK®
NCCN FOUNDATION
Guiding Treatment. Changing Lives.

NCCN Guidelines for Patients are supported by funding from the NCCN Foundation®

NCCN Foundation gratefully acknowledges the following corporate supporters for helping to make available these NCCN Guidelines for Patients: Karyopharm Therapeutics and Servier.

NCCN independently adapts, updates, and hosts the NCCN Guidelines for Patients. Our corporate supporters do not participate in the development of the NCCN Guidelines for Patients and are not responsible for the content and recommendations contained therein.

To make a gift or learn more, visit online or email

NCCNFoundation.org/donate

PatientGuidelines@NCCN.org

Contents

NCCN Foundation seeks to support the millions of patients and their families affected by a cancer diagnosis by funding and distributing NCCN Guidelines for Patients. NCCN Foundation is also committed to advancing cancer treatment by funding the nation's promising doctors at the center of innovation in cancer research. For more details and the full library of patient and caregiver resources, visit NCCN.org/patients.

National Comprehensive Cancer Network (NCCN) and NCCN Foundation
3025 Chemical Road, Suite 100, Plymouth Meeting, PA 19462 USA

1 About glioma

Being diagnosed with a brain tumor can be frightening and overwhelming. This book will help you make sense of all the information that's out there. It will also describe your options for treatment. Gliomas can be challenging to treat, but treatment is improving.

What is a glioma?

A glioma is a type of tumor that grows in the brain. A tumor is an abnormal growth of cells. Gliomas develop from certain brain cells called glial cells. Glial cells support the function of nerve cells (neurons) in the central nervous system (the brain and the spinal cord). Many types of tumors can occur in the central nervous system. Only those that start as glial cells become gliomas.

Gliomas are the most common type of malignant (cancerous) brain tumor in adults. Gliomas can happen at any age but occur more often in adults than in children. Gliomas start in the brain or sometimes the spinal cord. But they rarely spread to another area of the body.

What makes gliomas so complicated is that they invade and blend into the normal parts of the brain. So gliomas can be very difficult to treat without harming the healthy parts of the brain.

Normal cells vs. cancer cells

Normal cells follow the body's rules. Normal cells increase in number only when they're needed, and they die when they're old or damaged.

Cancer cells don't follow the rules. Cancer cells can multiply quickly and avoid dying. Cancer cells can crowd out normal cells and take their place. Eventually this damages the body and often results in symptoms.

What causes a glioma?

No one knows exactly what causes most brain tumors, including gliomas.

What experts do know is that brain tumors often start with an abnormality (mutation) in certain cells. This abnormality causes these cells to grow out of control (become cancerous). This type of mutation happens on its own. It's not typically passed down in families (hereditary mutation).

Gliomas occur in both children and adults. This book discusses gliomas only in adults.

Are there types of gliomas?

There are several types of glioma tumors. The 3 most common types are astrocytomas, oligodendrogliomas, and glioblastomas. They're made of different kinds of glial cells.

- **Astrocytomas** look like star-shaped glial cells called astrocytes. The main job of astrocytes is to maintain the chemical environment that allows communication between nerve cells.
- **Oligodendrogliomas** look like oligodendrocytes, which are glial cells that protect electrical signaling in nerve cells.
- **Glioblastomas** come from precursor cells that develop into cells like astrocytes and oligodendrocytes. Glioblastomas are the most destructive and dangerous type of glioma tumor.

Besides tumor type, gliomas are also categorized by grade. The grade indicates how fast the tumor is likely to grow. A low-grade glioma usually grows slowly while a high-grade glioma often grows rapidly.

Although it helps to put gliomas into categories, it's important to note that each glioma has its own molecular characteristics and behavior. That also means that each person's glioma is unique. So your progress and experience will be unique to you.

Gliomas often occur in the upper part of the brain where they can disrupt important brain functions.

Few gliomas in adults have distinct and well-defined edges like the one in this illustration. Most gliomas blend deeply into normal brain tissue and have vague borders. This makes them very difficult to remove entirely. When the tumor is removed, some tumor cells must be left behind to avoid damaging nearby brain tissue.

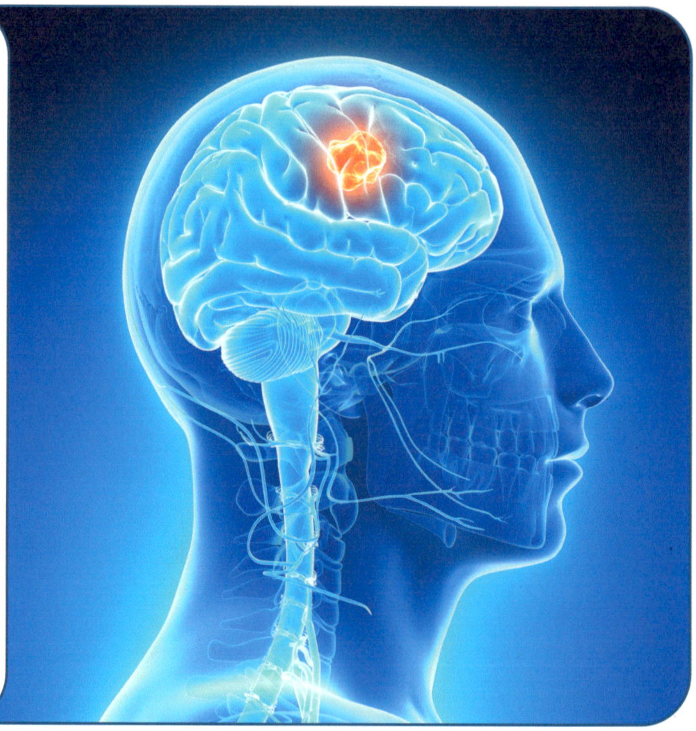

How are gliomas diagnosed?

A glioma is often found when it starts causing symptoms. A symptom is a problem or feeling that may be a sign of disease. Gliomas cause symptoms when they put pressure on the brain or invade brain tissue. Some people have many symptoms while others don't have any. Common symptoms of gliomas include:

- Unusual or frequent headaches
- Seizures
- Changes in personality or mood
- Nausea and vomiting
- Difficulty speaking or swallowing
- Muscle weakness
- Difficulty with walking, balance, or coordination

Symptoms provide clues that something is wrong. But they don't provide enough information to identify a specific illness. Different tests, physical exams, and surgical procedures are required to diagnose a glioma.

If these tests show that you have a glioma, your care team will discuss your treatment options with you. If possible, seek care at a center with experience in treating brain tumors.

Diagnosis vs. prognosis

What's the difference between your diagnosis and your prognosis? These two words sound alike but they're very different.

Diagnosis: The identification of an illness based on tests. The diagnosis names what illness you have.

Prognosis: The likely course and outcome of a disease. The prognosis predicts how your disease will turn out.

Can gliomas be cured?

Most gliomas are not curable, but they are usually treatable. Treatment can slow down the tumor's growth for a period of time, reduce its symptoms, and prolong life. The main treatments for a glioma are surgery, radiation therapy, and chemotherapy. These are often combined with one another for more complete treatment.

Another option to consider is participating in a clinical trial for a potential new treatment.

Treatment may be able to stop the glioma from growing and keep it stabilized for a time. This may last for months or years. However, even with the best treatment, gliomas usually grow back eventually. So periodic follow-up visits and additional rounds of treatment are recommended.

It's true that gliomas are eventually fatal for most patients. Many people diagnosed with a glioma have a difficult road ahead. Still, there's hope. New therapies designed to treat specific types of gliomas are currently being studied in clinical trials. The number of these trials has increased in recent years, offering more hope to people living with this disease.

Also, be aware that survival statistics come from research done several (or many) years ago. Those statistics may not reflect the improvements offered by today's diagnostic tests and treatments.

What's next?

This chapter provided a brief introduction on gliomas. The next chapter explains the tests needed to diagnose and monitor this disease.

A message to caregivers and loved ones

This book is for you, too. This book will help you understand this disease and the challenges it presents. People with tumors in the central nervous system (the brain and spinal cord) commonly develop problems with brain function. This can show itself in multiple ways, such as slower thinking, memory loss, difficulty moving or walking, trouble speaking, inability to do everyday activities, changes in behavior, losing one's sense of self, and other problems.

Helping a person with a brain tumor can be challenging and time-consuming. You may be providing physical, mental, emotional, and hands-on support. You may be taking the patient to appointments, helping to lessen side effects, and even assisting with treatment decisions. Gather as much help as you can. Start with the online resources listed in the back of this book.

Key points

- Gliomas develop from brain cells called glial cells. Glial cells support the function of nerve cells in the brain and the spinal cord.
- Gliomas can disrupt the brain's ability to function properly.
- Gliomas can be difficult to treat because they frequently invade and blend into the normal parts of the brain.
- What causes gliomas is unknown. What is known is that gliomas often start with an abnormality (mutation) that makes glial cells grow out of control.
- The 3 most common types of glioma tumors are astrocytomas, oligodendrogliomas, and glioblastomas.
- Several different tests and procedures are usually needed to diagnose a glioma.
- Gliomas can be treated but usually return at some point.

"Don't Google your diagnosis and assume that statistics define your life! Every person's brain tumor story and situation is different."

2

Glioma testing

Different tests are needed to find out whether you have a glioma and what type it is. Testing also suggests what kind of therapy is most appropriate for you.

You'll need a variety of tests to diagnose a brain tumor and to make a treatment plan. (If you've already had testing and received a glioma diagnosis, you can turn to Chapter 3 to read about your treatment options.)

Testing begins with an examination of your general health and an evaluation of your symptoms. Bring someone with you to listen, ask questions, and write down the answers.

Health and symptoms

Your care team needs to have all of your health information. They'll ask you about any health problems and treatments you've had. Be prepared to talk about any illness or injury you've had and when it happened. Tell your care team about any symptoms you have.

Symptoms

Each part of the brain has its own job to do. Different parts of the brain manage different parts of the body. Symptoms occur when an area of the brain doesn't work properly.

Symptoms are often related to the location of the tumor in the brain as well as the size of the tumor. Symptoms develop as the glioma grows against, or weaves itself into, a part of the brain. This growth can cause swelling (edema) in the brain tissue around the tumor. Sometimes a tumor blocks the flow of fluid (cerebrospinal fluid) in and around the brain.

Some people with low-grade gliomas never have symptoms. Low-grade gliomas generally grow slowly and can develop for years before they're diagnosed. High-grade gliomas can cause a range of symptoms. These gliomas can grow quickly, developing in months or weeks. However, symptoms can also be caused by medical problems other than tumors. So for the most accurate diagnosis, be sure to tell your provider and care team about any and all symptoms you're having, even if the symptoms seem unrelated.

Common symptoms include:

- **Headaches** – Headaches are very common and often the first symptom in people with a glioma. Headaches can be worse in the morning, wake you up in the middle of the night, and occur with nausea and vomiting.
- **Seizures** – Seizures are also frequent in people with brain tumors. Seizures are often an early sign of a glioma, especially in low-grade gliomas.
- **Fatigue** – Fatigue is another common symptom of a glioma. Fatigue can be debilitating, frequent, emotionally overwhelming, and not related to how much sleep you get or how much activity you do. However, physical activity or exercise can sometimes help.
- **Nausea and vomiting** – Nausea and vomiting can be caused by the tumor putting increased pressure on the brain.

- **Problems with thinking and speech** – Examples include confusion, memory loss, and speech difficulties.
- **Weakness or problems moving** – People with a brain tumor may have muscle weakness on one side of the body, or difficulty with walking or balance.
- **Changes in personality or mood** – Changes in behavior, mood, and personality can occur in people whose tumors are located in parts of the brain that control mood and personality.

Other symptoms also sometimes occur. Gliomas can cause vision problems such as blurred vision, double vision, or loss of peripheral (side) vision. Sensory disturbances include numbness, tingling, or burning sensations often on one side of the body. And high-grade gliomas are linked to blood clots in the legs and the lungs, which can cause leg swelling, chest pain, and shortness of breath.

If you have any of these symptoms, your provider may want to take a closer look. This is where imaging comes in, which is discussed on the next page.

Areas of the brain and their functions

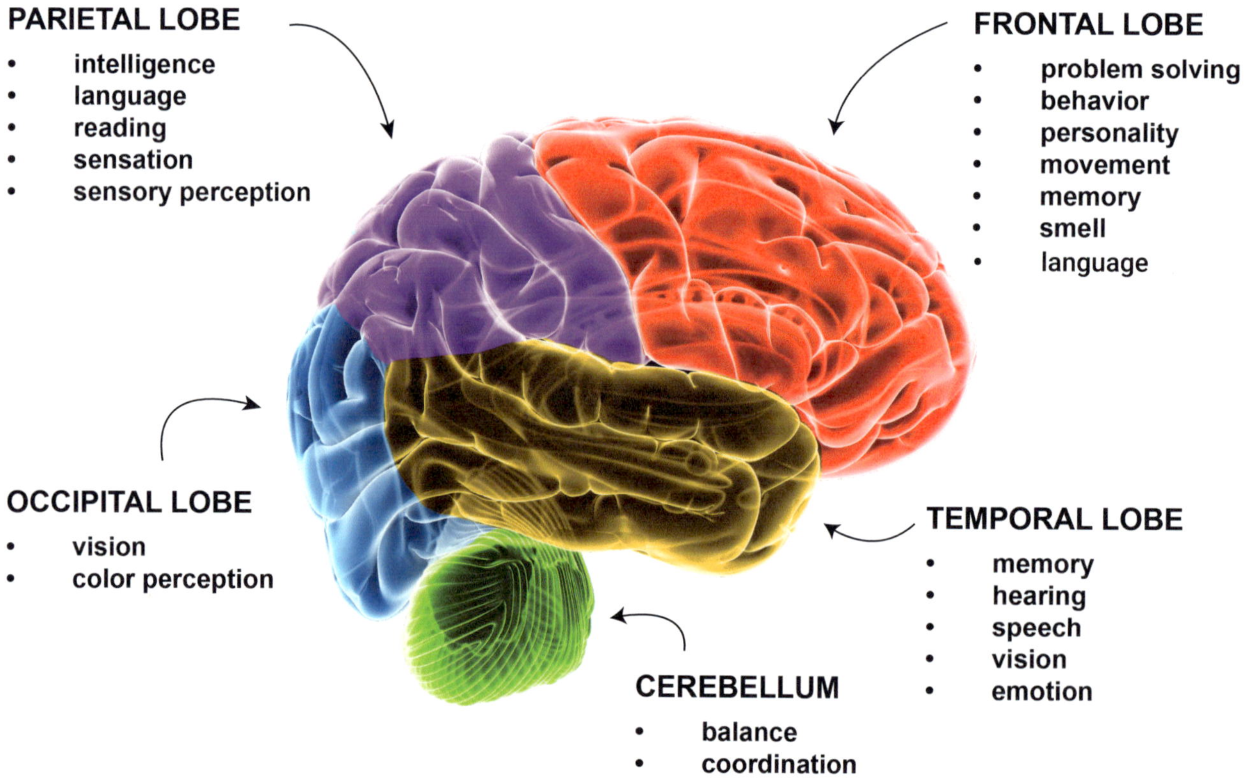

Neurological exam

A neurological exam involves some simple tests to check your alertness, thinking, balance, coordination, reflexes, strength, hearing, and senses of touch and smell. You may also have an eye exam to check the health of the nerves in the back of your eyes.

Performance status

Your team will want to know how well you can do ordinary day-to-day activities—like working, taking a walk, climbing stairs, cooking dinner, carrying laundry, or taking a bath or shower. This evaluation is called performance status. The more activities you can do, the better your performance status. Your care team uses this evaluation to get a sense of the level of treatment you may be able to handle and whether you may be eligible for a clinical trial.

Imaging

If you have signs or symptoms of a brain tumor, your care team will want to try to find it and see what it looks like. Imaging tests are used to make pictures (images) of the insides of your body. The images can reveal a tumor's location, size, and other features.

MRI

Magnetic resonance imaging (MRI) is the most useful imaging test for identifying a glioma. MRI scans are good at showing the soft tissues, including the brain, as well as other details that help plan surgery.

> **"Fatigue is more than just being tired. It can be physical, cognitive, or emotional. It can be created from external sources, such as noise, or internal sources, such as medication, not eating properly, or not getting enough exercise."**

MRI uses a magnetic field and radio waves to take pictures of the inside of the body. During an MRI, you'll lie on a table that slides into the scanning machine. (An open MRI scanner may be an option at some health care centers.) It's important to lie still during the test to get the best pictures. You may be given a padded head brace or other devices to help you stay motionless. The machine makes loud noises but you can wear earplugs and listen to music.

You'll have multiple MRI tests throughout diagnosis and treatment. MRI is also used after treatment to see how well the treatment worked. You'll have more MRIs during follow-up to watch for any recurrence or new growth.

CT

If MRI is unavailable or not recommended for you, you might have a computed tomography (CT or CAT) scan instead. A CT scan uses x-rays to take many images of your body from different angles. A computer then combines the pictures to make a 3D image.

After imaging

After the MRI or CT scan, your images will be studied by a radiologist, an expert in analyzing images of the nervous system. The radiologist will convey the imaging results to your care team. This information helps your team plan what the next steps of your care should be.

If your images seem to show a glioma, the next step may be a biopsy.

Biopsy

If imaging scans show something that may be a glioma, your care providers will usually want to take a sample and evaluate it. A surgical procedure that removes a small piece of tissue for testing is called a biopsy. Getting a biopsy of a tumor is the only way to get an accurate diagnosis of your condition. A biopsy also gives your care team clues on how to treat your tumor.

A surgical procedure called a **resection** does double duty as both a biopsy and a treatment. In a resection, your neurosurgeon will attempt to remove the entire tumor or as much of the tumor as safely possible. Removing the tumor could relieve symptoms and help you live longer. Also, a large sample of the tumor can give the most complete pathology results.

Sometimes a resection isn't possible. This happens when the glioma is in a difficult place to reach or is located in a vital part of the brain. In these cases, your provider will schedule a standard biopsy.

There are 2 types of standard biopsies for gliomas: stereotactic biopsy and open biopsy.

Stereotactic biopsy

This is a very precise procedure that's often used when a brain tumor is in a hard-to-reach or vital area. It aims to remove only enough of the tumor to make a diagnosis.

A stereotactic biopsy is done by a neurosurgeon in an operating room. First, you'll be fitted with a frame or several tiny markers around your head to aid the surgery. Next, you'll be given anesthesia to go to sleep. A small area of your hair will be trimmed down to the scalp.

The neurosurgeon will then make a little opening in your skull and insert a thin, hollow needle into the brain to remove a sliver of the tumor. A computerized navigation system, connected to MRI or CT imaging, will allow the surgeon to target and remove the sample with a high degree of precision. After removal, the opening in your scalp will be closed with sutures. You may be able to go home the next day.

Open biopsy

Like a resection, an open biopsy is a surgical procedure that involves making a small opening in the skull (craniotomy).

First, you'll be given anesthesia that will let you sleep through the procedure. Your neurosurgeon will cut open a section of your scalp and then remove a piece of skull bone. Using small surgical knives and other special instruments, the neurosurgeon will carefully remove a piece or pieces of the tumor. The segment of skull bone will be replaced and the incision will be sewn up.

Lab testing

After either type of biopsy, the tissue sample will be sent to a laboratory for analysis. A specialist called a neuropathologist will examine the tissue under a microscope.

Sometimes, the sample is taken straight to the neuropathologist while you're still in the operating room. The neuropathologist will perform an analysis right away and send the results back to the neurosurgeon.

The results will say whether the tumor is malignant (cancerous) or benign (not cancerous). The results may also include the preliminary diagnosis, including the type and grade of the glioma. Knowing the preliminary diagnosis during your surgery helps the neurosurgeon to decide how much of the tumor to remove.

The neuropathologist will also do molecular (genetic) testing, which indicates the type and growth rate of your glioma and other specific features. All this information will help your treatment team figure out the best treatment plan for you.

If your hospital or medical center doesn't have a neuropathologist, you can ask to have your biopsy sent to one.

Stereotactic biopsy

A stereotactic biopsy is needed to diagnose a glioma tumor. In this procedure, a thin, hollow needle is inserted into the brain to remove a sliver of the tumor. The sample is sent to a lab to be tested for cancer cells.

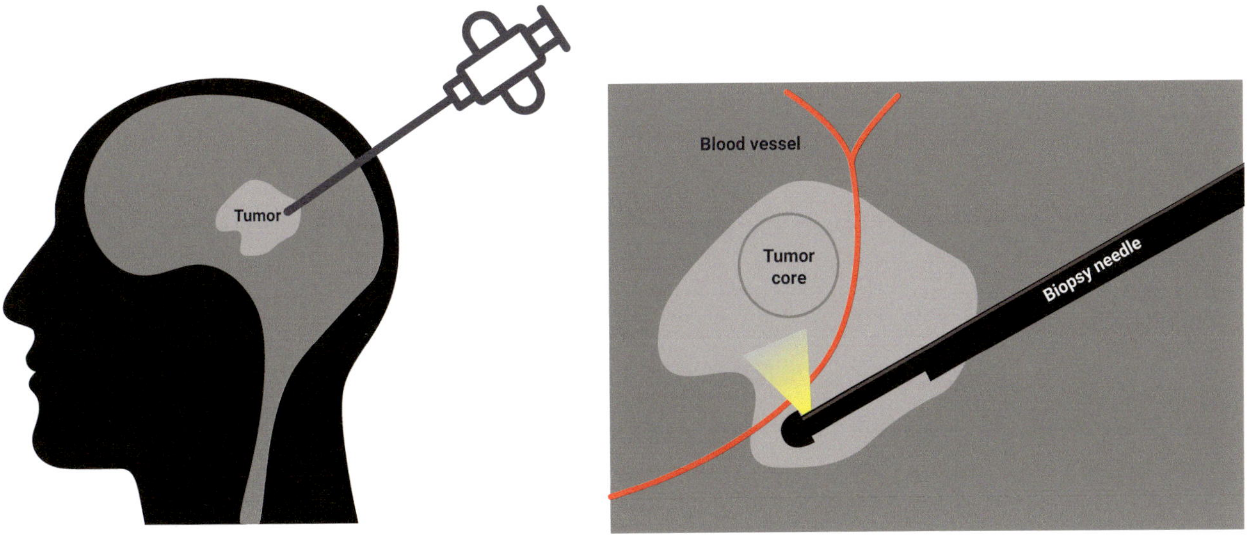

Your tumor type

If molecular testing was performed on your biopsy sample, the pathology report should reveal your tumor type. It's important to identify the exact type of tumor you have to predict the course of your disease and plan your treatment.

There are 3 ways to classify a glioma:

- **Histology** – The first way to classify the tumor is by looking at it under a microscope. This is called histology. For instance, a glioma with cells that look like astrocytes is likely to be an astrocytoma.
- **Grade** – Another way to classify a tumor is by grade, which is a rating of how abnormal its cells are. The more abnormal its cells, the faster and farther the tumor is likely to grow.
- **Biomarkers** – A glioma is also identified by its biomarkers. A biomarker is a molecular characteristic such as a genetic mutation. Each type of glioma has its own biomarker or set of biomarkers. For example, an astrocytoma may have a mutation in the *IDH* gene. So it would be called an astrocytoma *IDH*-mutant.

When these 3 classifications are put together, it provides a full description of the glioma. For example, an "astrocytoma *IDH*-mutant grade 2" names its cell type (astrocytoma), its biomarker (*IDH*-mutant), and its growth rate (grade 2).

Let's look at each of these classifications in turn.

Histology

Histology means evaluating the structure of cells or tissues under a microscope. A neuropathologist does a histologic analysis when inspecting tissue from a biopsy. The neuropathologist will examine the tumor cells to classify the disease. The neuropathologist's report will state if the tumor started in the central nervous system or elsewhere. If the tumor is a glioma, the cell type will be noted in the report.

The types of gliomas are named after the glial cells that they resemble. The neuropathologist can see this under the microscope. For example, an astrocytoma looks like cells called astrocytes. And an oligodendroglioma looks like oligodendrocytes.

"Brain tumors are insidious because the symptom burden can feel like an attack on the very nature of the self, including personality changes, language and memory impairment, physical impairment, and poor prognosis."

Grade

Another way that gliomas are classified is by grade. The grade indicates how quickly the glioma is likely to grow and spread. Tumors are graded from 1 to 4 based mostly on how much the tumor cells look like normal cells. Low-grade gliomas include grades 1 and 2. High-grade gliomas include grades 3 and 4. Grades are used to predict the outlook (prognosis) of the tumor and to plan treatment.

- **Grade 1** tumors grow slowly and are usually benign. Many people with grade 1 gliomas can be treated with surgery alone. But if the tumor grows back, additional therapy may be given. Grade 1 gliomas are more common in children than in adults.
- **Grade 2** tumor cells look somewhat abnormal. These tumors grow slowly and can invade normal tissue. They may not grow back for many years. But when they do, they usually come back as a higher-grade glioma.
- **Grade 3** tumor cells don't look much like normal cells. They quickly increase in number and invade nearby tissue. All high-grade tumors (grades 3 and 4) require additional therapy—like radiation and chemotherapy—after surgery.
- **Grade 4** tumor cells look very abnormal. These tumors grow and spread very quickly. Glioblastomas are the most common grade 4 gliomas.

Biomarkers

The neuropathologist also tests the tissue sample for specific biomarkers. Biomarker tests provide more details about the glioma tumor. A biomarker is something found in the body that's a sign of a condition, disease, or abnormality.

In cancer care, biomarker testing looks for changes in genes, proteins, and other markers. Many of these changes are mutations. A mutation is an abnormal change in your DNA—your body's genetic instructions. A mutation can disrupt how some cells behave, which can cause diseases like cancer.

Biomarker testing can improve the accuracy of your diagnosis as well as fine-tune your treatment options. If testing detects a certain mutation, you might be able to receive treatment that's targeted more precisely to your glioma. Right now, only a few targeted treatments are available for very specific kinds of glioma. But researchers are working on hundreds of clinical trials to find more.

The following biomarkers aren't the only biomarkers of gliomas, but they're the most commonly tested. Finding these biomarkers (or not finding them) can provide specific information about your glioma. **See Guide 1** on the next page.

Ask what biomarker testing is available for your glioma. Some hospitals and treatment centers aren't able to provide a full range of biomarker tests. But you can request your tissue to be sent to another lab for further testing.

What's next?

After you've been diagnosed and have gone through further testing, your treatment team will discuss your results with you. You'll also talk about your options for treatment based on your test results. The next chapter discusses the different options for treating gliomas.

> **"Ask as many questions as possible during appointments and bring a family member with you to take notes."**

Guide 1
Biomarkers identify specific gliomas

Each type of glioma is identified by the biomarkers it has (✓) and those it doesn't have (✗).

	Oligodendroglioma grade 2 or 3	Astrocytoma grade 2 or 3	Astrocytoma grade 4	Glioblastoma grade 4
***IDH* mutation**	✓	✓	✓	✗
1p/19q co-deletion	✓	✗	✗	
***ATRX* mutation**	✗	✓	✓	
***TERT* promoter mutation**	✓	✗	✗	✓
7 gain/ 10 loss				✓
***EGFR* mutation**				✓
CDKN2A/B		✗	✓	

Key points

- The best way to diagnose a glioma is with a surgical biopsy or a resection.
- Symptoms of a brain tumor are related to its location as well as its size. Symptoms develop as the glioma grows against and into the brain tissue.
- Imaging tests are used to help with diagnosis, treatment planning, and assessing treatment results. Imaging scans can identify a tumor's location, size, and other features.
- The most common imaging test for glioma is an MRI, or magnetic resonance imaging.
- A neuropathologist will inspect a tissue sample from your biopsy under a microscope. This can confirm whether you have a glioma and what type it may be.
- Low-grade tumors grow very slowly and may not come back for years after surgery. High-grade tumor cells look very different from normal cells and typically grow very quickly.
- Biomarker testing analyzes your glioma for abnormal changes in genes, proteins, and other markers. Biomarker testing is needed for a final diagnosis as well as for fine-tuning your treatment plan.

share with us.

Take our survey and help make the NCCN Guidelines for Patients better for everyone!

NCCN.org/patients/comments

3

Overview of glioma treatments

Treatment options vary depending on the cell type, grade, size, and location of the tumor. Your care team will explain the benefits and risks of all your available options.

There are many ways to try to treat a glioma, but none are perfect. The most common treatment options include surgery, radiation therapy, chemotherapy, or a combination of these.

The first treatment is usually surgery to remove as much of the tumor as possible or to biopsy the tumor.

Next, you may have radiation therapy and chemotherapy to destroy the tumor cells left behind. For example, surgery may take away the majority of the tumor. Then radiation therapy can attack what's left of the tumor cells. **See Guide 2.**

Surgery

The first aim of surgery is to safely take out as much of the tumor as possible (resection). In general, the more tumor that's removed, the better your prognosis. Surgery may also relieve pressure inside the skull and lessen seizures or other symptoms that are hard to control.

Another aim of surgery is to confirm the diagnosis. During tumor surgery, tissue is removed from the tumor and tested to confirm whether it's a glioma and what type it is.

A neurosurgeon (an expert in surgery of the nervous system) will perform your surgery. Deciding which procedure to perform is a complex and difficult decision. Should it be a resection, a partial resection, or a biopsy? Is surgery even possible? Not all people with gliomas will be able to have surgery.

Guide 2
Basic treatment plan for most gliomas

Main treatment	• Surgery to remove all or most of the tumor
Additional treatments	• Clinical trial • Radiation therapy • Chemotherapy

The neurosurgeon will talk with your multidisciplinary team, and they'll consider many factors:

- Your age
- Your performance status
- Expected tumor type and grade
- How close the tumor is to "eloquent" areas of the brain
- Whether the surgery might relieve pressure on the brain
- Whether the tumor can be easily and safely removed
- The time since your last surgery (for people with a recurrent glioma)

Eloquent areas of the brain are those that control important functions like speech, vision, hearing, and movement. Damage to an eloquent area can impair the related function in the body. This is why surgeons must be careful about how much tissue they remove.

What is awake surgery?

You may need to be awake during part of the operation if your tumor is located near parts of the brain that control senses, movement, or speech. The neurosurgeon will stimulate these functional areas while asking you questions.

You'll be conscious but given local anesthesia and a light sedative so that you won't feel pain.

To locate areas for movement, the surgeon may ask you to wiggle your toes or your fingers. To identify language areas, you may be asked to count out loud or perform other speech tests. This lets the surgeon know what tissue can be taken out and what needs to stay. After the tumor tissue is removed, you'll be sedated for the rest of the operation.

Resection

Resection is a major surgery that removes a large piece of tissue. In a full resection (also called a gross total resection), the neurosurgeon removes all of the tumor that can be detected with imaging. A partial resection removes part of the tumor. A full resection offers a better chance of fewer symptoms and longer life.

You may need to be awake during part of the operation so that the key brain areas can be found. You'll still be given some anesthesia to help you relax during an awake surgery.

The surgeon will use a small drill to remove a piece of your skull (craniotomy). A cut into your brain may be needed to reach the tumor.

This is a delicate and precise operation. Surgeons often use computers programmed with MRI or CT scans of your tumor to guide the surgery. This technology serves as a GPS for your brain. It helps the surgeon to precisely locate and carefully remove as much tumor as possible without removing nearby brain tissue.

After the tumor is removed, the small piece of your skull will be replaced, and you'll be given time to recover. You'll have another MRI or CT the day after the surgery to confirm how much of the tumor was removed.

For most gliomas, there are microscopic tumor cells that can't be seen, even with imaging systems like MRI, in the tissue outside of the tumor. So some tumor cells are almost always left behind after the tumor is removed.

Radiation therapy

You may be given radiation therapy after you recover from surgery to try to destroy any glioma cells that remain. Radiation therapy is used to treat both fully resected and partially resected tumors. A radiation oncologist—an expert in using radiation to treat cancer—will manage your radiation treatment.

Radiation therapy focuses high-energy rays on tumor cells. The rays are delivered to the tumor area to damage the DNA inside the tumor cells. This either kills the tumor cells or stops new tumor cells from being made. You won't see, hear, or feel the radiation. It passes through your skin and other tissues to reach the tumor.

"Go to a hospital that specializes in brain tumors."

Depending on the type of glioma, radiation may be delivered to the tumor plus some tissue around it that contains both tumor cells and normal cells. Because radiation can harm normal cells, your radiation oncologist will use methods that avoid and lessen the radiation applied to normal brain tissues. Your radiation plan will be tailored to you, your tumor, and your brain.

Radiation therapy

To receive radiation therapy, you may be fitted with a mesh mask to help hold your head still. While you stay still during treatment, the radiation machine moves around you.

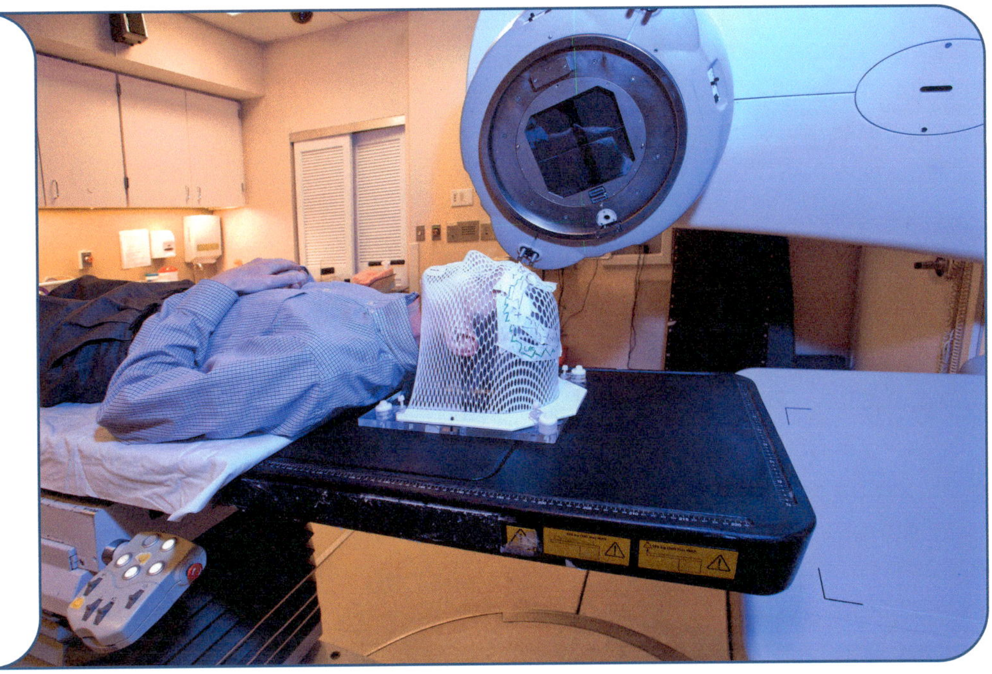

Receiving radiation

During treatment, you'll lie on the treatment table and be told how to get into the position needed for treatment. You must remain completely motionless during radiation treatment. You'll be fitted with a special head mask to help you hold still. Other devices may also be used to help you to stay still during radiation therapy.

The total dose of radiation is spread out over a number of treatments (fractions). The number of treatments varies among patients. Treatments are usually given once a day, up to 5 days a week, for 2 to 6 weeks. One session takes about 15 to 30 minutes. This includes only a few minutes of actual radiation time. Your radiation oncologist will see you every week to review how you're doing.

Side effects of radiation

Your radiation oncologist will discuss the possible side effects of radiation. Side effects from radiation therapy differ among people. Factors like tumor type, tumor location, radiation dose, length of treatment, and other factors all play a role. Side effects are cumulative, meaning they intensify over the course of treatment.

The most common side effect of radiation is tiredness despite sleep (fatigue). You may also have hair loss or irritation on your scalp where treatment was applied. Other side effects of radiation include swelling (which may feel like pressure inside your head), headache, and sometimes nausea or loss of appetite. Rare side effects include seizures, hearing loss, speech or memory problems, and worsening of symptoms you already had before treatment started. Possible long-term side effects include a decrease in mental functioning. Your multidisciplinary team will work with you to help with these problems.

These aren't the only side effects of radiation. Ask your treatment team for a complete list of common and rare side effects. If a side effect bothers you, tell your treatment team. There may be ways to help you feel better. There are also ways to prevent some side effects.

Chemotherapy

Chemotherapy uses drugs to damage and destroy rapidly dividing cells throughout the body. Because tumor cells divide and multiply rapidly, they're a good target for chemotherapy. Chemotherapy can harm healthy cells, too. That's why chemotherapy can cause side effects.

Receiving chemotherapy

A single chemotherapy drug or a combination of drugs can be used for treatment. Temozolomide (Temodar) is a standard single chemotherapy drug for glioma. A combination of drugs is sometimes chosen because these drugs work better when they're used together. A common drug combination for glioma treatment is procarbazine, lomustine, and vincristine (or PCV).

Your neuro-oncologist or medical oncologist will discuss your chemotherapy options with you.

Chemotherapy is given in cycles. One cycle involves a few treatment days followed by several days for recovery. The cycles vary in length depending on which drugs are used. Common cycles are 14, 21, or 28 days long. Having chemotherapy in cycles gives your body a chance to recover after receiving the treatment. If you're going to have chemotherapy, ask your medical oncologist how many cycles and days of treatment there will be within a cycle.

Some chemotherapy drugs are given through an intravenous (IV) infusion into a vein in your arm or another part of your body. Other chemotherapy drugs (like temozolomide) can be taken as a pill.

One chemotherapy drug, carmustine (Gliadel), is given as a "wafer" implant and must be placed inside the brain at the time of surgery. Each wafer is about the size of a dime. Up to 8 wafers may be used. They're placed into the brain during total resection, in the space where the tumor had been. The wafers treat the leftover tumor cells in the surrounding tissue. The wafers dissolve over time, letting out chemotherapy little by little. Be aware that receiving this treatment may disqualify you from joining a clinical trial.

Chemotherapy is usually given in combination with radiation therapy. The timing of chemotherapy is based on the tumor's grade and rate of growth, your health and performance status, the success of surgical tumor removal, and other factors.

Side effects of chemotherapy

The side effects of chemotherapy depend on many things. These include the drug, the amount taken, the length of treatment, and the person. Some people have many side effects. Others have few.

Some side effects can be very serious. Others are not serious but are still unpleasant. Most side effects appear while you're undergoing treatment and then stop after treatment is over. Other side effects are long-term or may even appear years later.

Common side effects of chemotherapy include low blood cell counts, not feeling hungry, nausea, vomiting, diarrhea, hair loss, fatigue, and mouth sores. Ask your neuro-oncologist or medical oncologist which drugs cause which side effects. Medication is available to manage or prevent some side effects. To learn about preventing and managing nausea and vomiting, read the *NCCN Guidelines for Patients: Nausea and Vomiting* available at NCCN.org/patientguidelines and on the NCCN Patient Guides for Cancer app.

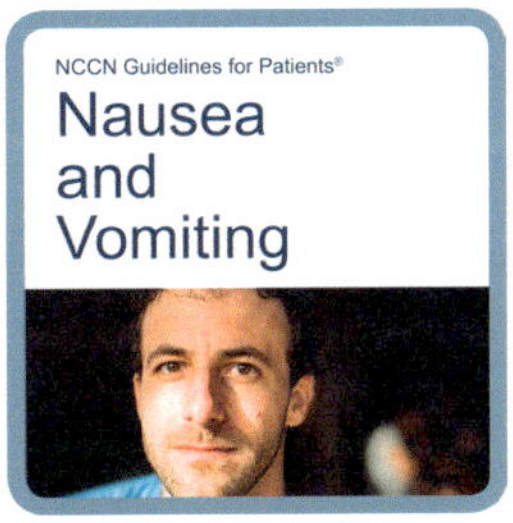

Not all side effects of chemotherapy are listed here. Ask your team for a complete list of common and rare side effects, and what treatments are available.

Alternating electric field therapy

Alternating electric field therapy is a treatment that uses low-intensity energy to stop tumor cells from multiplying. It's also called tumor treating fields (TTFields). This treatment is an option for certain people with newly diagnosed or recurrent glioblastomas.

Here's the idea behind this therapy: Tumor cells multiply by dividing into more tumor cells. Electromagnetic TTFields disrupt this replication process. The energy is "tuned" specifically to glioblastoma cells to interfere with their cell division. TTFields destroy newly dividing tumor cells but don't affect healthy cells.

The TTFields device (called Optune Gio) looks something like a swim cap connected with wires to a carry-along battery pack. The electric field energy is distributed through electrodes attached to several patches that safely adhere to your scalp. Because the patches need to be placed on skin, your hair will be shaved. The electrodes are linked to an energy-producing device and a battery you carry with you. You wear it at home and when going out. You can wear a wig, a scarf, or a hat over it if you want.

The treatment is intended to be used for at least 18 hours a day for at least 4 weeks. The most common side effect is skin irritation.

Alternating electric field therapy

Alternating electric field therapy—also called tumor treating fields (TTFields)—uses low-intensity energy to stop tumor cells from multiplying. Electromagnetic field energy is distributed through electrodes attached to four patches taped to your scalp. The energy is "tuned" to glioblastoma cells and interferes with their cell division. TTFields destroy newly dividing tumor cells but don't affect healthy cells.

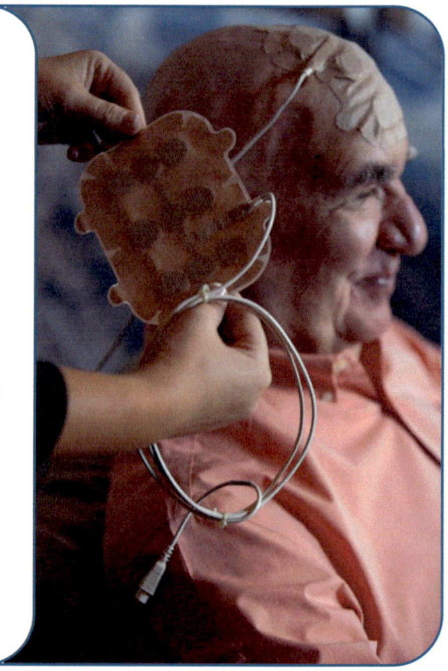

Targeted therapy

Targeted therapy drugs attack certain parts of tumor cells to slow their growth and spread. Because targeted therapy is aimed only at tumor cells not healthy cells, it doesn't have the same side effects as standard chemotherapy.

At this time, only a few targeted therapy drugs are available for gliomas. Also, they're only effective against gliomas that multiply or spread through the specific enzyme, protein, or other molecule that they target. For example, a BRAF inhibitor only works against tumor cells that have a mutation in the *BRAF* gene.

Observation

The recommended treatment for most gliomas is surgical removal (resection). However, observation may be a better or safer option for some people. Observation means your treatment team will check on your condition using regular tests over a period of time. No treatment is given unless symptoms appear or your condition changes.

Supportive care

Supportive care (also called palliative care) is health care for the symptoms of cancer and the side effects of cancer treatment. Supportive care is appropriate for anyone, regardless of age, cancer stage, or the need for other therapies.

For more information about supportive care, *see Chapter 7*.

Clinical trials

NCCN experts recommend that everyone with a glioma consider joining a clinical trial for treatment.

A clinical trial is a type of medical research study. Clinical trials are a key way to assess new treatment approaches. After being developed and tested in a laboratory, potential new ways of fighting cancer need to be studied in people. If found to be safe and effective in a clinical trial, a drug, device, or treatment approach may be approved by the U.S. Food and Drug Administration (FDA).

Talk to your treatment team about whether a clinical trial makes sense for you. Everyone with cancer should carefully consider all the treatment options available for their type of cancer, including standard treatments and clinical trials.

Who can enroll?

Every clinical trial has rules for joining, called eligibility criteria. The rules may be about age, cancer type and stage, treatment history, or general health. These requirements ensure that participants are alike in certain ways and that the trial is as safe as possible for the participants.

Informed consent

Clinical trials are managed by a group of experts called a research team. The research team will review the study with you in detail, including its purpose and the risks and benefits of joining. All of this information is also provided in an informed consent form. This is an agreement that confirms you've been fully told about your part in the trial. Read the form carefully and ask questions before signing it. Take time to discuss it with family, friends, or other people you trust. Keep in mind that you can leave and seek treatment outside of the clinical trial at any time.

Start the conversation

Don't wait for your treatment team to bring up clinical trials. Start the conversation and learn about all your treatment options. If you find a study that you may be eligible for, ask your treatment team if you meet the requirements. Try not to be discouraged if you cannot join. New clinical trials are always becoming available.

Frequently asked questions

There are many myths and misconceptions surrounding clinical trials. The possible benefits and risks are not well understood by many with cancer.

Will I get a placebo?

Placebos (inactive versions of real medicines) are almost never used alone in cancer clinical trials. It's common to receive either a placebo with a standard treatment or a new drug with a standard treatment. You'll be informed if a placebo is part of a clinical trial before you enroll.

Are clinical trials free?

There's no fee to enroll in a clinical trial. The study sponsor pays for research-related costs, including the study drug. You may, however, have costs indirectly related to the trial, such as the cost of transportation or childcare due to extra appointments and the costs of routine patient care during the trial. Depending on the trial, you may continue to receive standard cancer care. The standard therapy is billed to—and often covered by—insurance. You're responsible for copays and any costs for this care that aren't covered by your insurance.

Finding a clinical trial

In the United States

NCCN Cancer Centers
NCCN.org/cancercenters

The National Cancer Institute (NCI)
cancer.gov/about-cancer/treatment/clinical-trials/search

Worldwide

The U.S. National Library of Medicine (NLM)
clinicaltrials.gov

Need help finding a clinical trial?

NCI's Cancer Information Service (CIS)
1.800.4.CANCER (1.800.422.6237)
cancer.gov/contact

What's next?

Now that you've been introduced to the various treatment options, the first step toward treatment is to come up with the best possible treatment plan. This plan involves many different health care providers.

Multidisciplinary care

During the course of your diagnosis and treatment, you'll be cared for by numerous doctors, specialists, and allied health providers.

These may include a neuro-oncologist, neurosurgeon, radiation oncologist, medical oncologist, neuropathologist, radiologist, ophthalmologist, nurses, primary care doctor, nurse practitioners, physician assistants, palliative care specialist, pain specialist, psychologist, social workers, nutritionist, and rehabilitation specialists like physical, occupational, and speech therapists.

When all these providers are working and communicating as a team to help you, it's called multidisciplinary care.

Your multidisciplinary care team should clearly discuss your care goals with you. Removing or reducing the size of your tumor is one goal of your team. But other goals could include improving your overall well-being, maintaining your ability to do day-to-day activities, reducing pain, getting good nutrition, and lowering stress and anxiety. Your multidisciplinary care team will meet to discuss your treatment and which options are best for you.

"Ask about clinical trials available to you and the services your hospital and other facilities provide to cancer patients, such as counseling, nutritional advice, meditation, physical therapy, palliative care, and integrative medicine. Don't be shy. Be your own advocate—or ask someone close to be one for you."

Ask who will coordinate your care and what efforts can be made to schedule appointments together.

The next chapter explains what your specific treatment may be if you have a low-grade glioma. The chapter after that discusses treatment details if you have a high-grade glioma.

Key points

- Surgery is performed to confirm the diagnosis and to remove as much of the tumor as possible.
- Radiation therapy uses high-energy rays to destroy tumor cells and stop them from increasing in number.
- Chemotherapy uses drugs to destroy tumor cells and stop them from increasing.
- Alternating electric field therapy uses low-intensity energy to stop tumor cells from multiplying.
- Targeted therapy is directed at a specific enzyme or another substance that is key to glioma cells.
- Clinical trials test new types of treatment. If an experimental treatment is proven to work well, it may be approved by the FDA and become widely available.
- Multidisciplinary care is when doctors, specialists, and allied health providers work and communicate as a team to provide expert diagnosis and treatment.

Create a medical binder

A medical binder or notebook is a great way to organize all of your records in one place.

Bring your binder to all your medical appointments. Records of your tests and images can be immensely helpful to your treatment team. Having all your records in one place will also be helpful when getting a second opinion.

✓ Include separate folders for your test results (blood, imaging, pathology, radiology, genetics), treatments, procedures, list of medications, and insurance forms. Organize items in the folders by date.

✓ Ask for CDs of your imaging scans and keep them in your binder, too.

✓ Use online patient portals to view your test results and other records. Download or print the records to add to your binder.

✓ Choose a binder that meets your needs. Consider a zipper pocket to include a pen, small calendar, and insurance cards.

✓ Add a section for questions and to take notes.

4

Treatment for low-grade glioma

Low-grade gliomas are less common than high-grade gliomas. They also have a better prognosis. Some low-grade gliomas eventually evolve into high-grade gliomas.

About low-grade gliomas

Low-grade gliomas include a variety of slow-growing grade 1 and grade 2 tumors. Low-grade gliomas typically occur in people between their teens and their 40s, but older adults can also get low-grade gliomas.

The most common symptom of low-grade gliomas is seizure (particularly in oligodendrogliomas). Other symptoms include headaches, muscle weakness, vision problems, and changes in mental function or behavior. However, many people with low-grade gliomas have no symptoms. Their tumors are often found during unrelated medical tests.

If your MRI scan shows what appears to be a low-grade glioma, the best possible plan is to remove the tumor surgically.

Tumor surgery

Although low-grade gliomas grow slowly, many eventually become high-grade gliomas. The main goal of treatment is to prevent or delay that from happening. The primary treatment for a low-grade glioma is surgery to remove the tumor (resection). Your treatment team may be able to tell from your MRI whether all of the tumor or part of the tumor can be removed.

- **Gross total resection** – A gross total resection is a surgical procedure that removes all, or nearly all, of the visible tumor. Ideally, the whole tumor can be removed. Removing the whole tumor is likely to help you live longer. It also helps to delay a low-grade glioma from becoming a high-grade glioma. Plus, it can further reduce seizures and other symptoms.
- **Partial resection** – Sometimes the tumor can't be removed entirely. Removing part of the tumor is called a partial resection. Your surgeon may recommend a second surgery later on to try to remove the whole tumor.

Pathology

Whether or not the whole tumor is removed, a sample of it will be sent to a neuropathologist. The neuropathologist will identify the type of glioma and test it for certain biomarkers. These results can also indicate the type of treatment you may need.

The most common low-grade gliomas in adults are astrocytomas and oligodendrogliomas.

Low-grade astrocytoma

Low-grade astrocytomas are slow-growing, diffuse grade 2 tumors. (Grade 1 astrocytomas usually occur only in children.) A diffuse (or infiltrative) tumor weaves into the surrounding normal brain tissue. This gives the tumor unclear, indistinct edges. As a result, a diffuse tumor is difficult to remove entirely by surgery.

Most diffuse astrocytomas in adults occur in the frontal or temporal lobes of the brain. Common symptoms are seizures and headaches. Other symptoms due to pressure on the brain are vision changes, nausea, and vomiting. Then again, a low-grade astrocytoma may cause no symptoms.

Biomarkers

Biomarkers help identify the glioma type and help guide treatment.

- ***IDH*** – *IDH* mutation is a key marker of astrocytomas. Also, some therapies may work relatively better in gliomas with an *IDH* mutation.

Treatment

The main treatment for a low-grade astrocytoma is a gross total resection to remove all the tumor or as much of it as possible.

After surgery, you'll be reevaluated for your next type of treatment (called adjuvant treatment). Your next treatment will be based on the risk of the tumor to regrow:

- **Low risk** – A person who is under 40 years old and has had a gross total resection usually has a low risk for the tumor to regrow quickly. Someone who has a lower risk tumor may be recommended for a clinical trial or kept under observation after surgery.
- **High risk** – A person who is over age 40 or has had a partial resection (or an open biopsy or a stereotactic biopsy) typically has a high risk for the tumor to regrow. Additional treatment for a person with high risk may involve a clinical trial. Otherwise, adjuvant treatment is usually radiation therapy followed by chemotherapy (PCV or temozolomide). Sometimes, radiation therapy is both combined with and followed by temozolomide chemotherapy.

There can be exceptions to these risk categories. Your care team will also consider the risks involved due to the tumor's size and whether you have any other gene mutations or neurological problems.

Also, people who are older or who have limited physical capability (low performance status) may not be able to handle such aggressive treatment. They might benefit from less intense therapy instead. Less intense adjuvant options include:

- Radiation therapy (possibly concentrated into a shorter period of time) with or without temozolomide chemotherapy
- Temozolomide chemotherapy only (which is preferred for people who have the *MGMT* promoter methylation biomarker)
- Supportive (palliative) care

Follow-up

After treatment, you'll have regular MRI or CT scans to make sure the tumor hasn't grown back. These will be scheduled for every 3 to 6 months at first, and then about every 6 months if the tumor remains stable. The scans will also monitor the health of your brain and identify any side effects of radiation therapy or chemotherapy.

Recurrence

The signs and symptoms of your astrocytoma may disappear for months or even several years after treatment. However, most grade 2 astrocytomas eventually evolve over time into higher-grade astrocytomas. To read about the recurrence of astrocytomas, *see Chapter 6.*

Low-grade oligodendroglioma

Low-grade oligodendrogliomas are slow-growing, grade 2 tumors. (There are no grade 1 oligodendrogliomas.) Oligodendrogliomas commonly develop in the frontal and temporal lobes of the brain. Tumors in these areas can result in symptoms such as seizures, headaches, weakness, and speech problems. The most common of these is seizure. About 3 in 5 people with an oligodendroglioma have a seizure before being diagnosed.

Biomarkers

Characteristic biomarkers of oligodendrogliomas are *IDH* mutation and 1p/19q co-deletion.

- ***IDH*** – An *IDH* mutation is found in all oligodendrogliomas.
- **1p/19q** – All oligodendrogliomas have 1p/19q co-deletion, which is linked to better results from chemotherapy.
- ***TERT* promoter** – A *TERT* promoter mutation, when it occurs along with *IDH* mutation and 1p/19q co-deletion, helps confirm the diagnosis of oligodendroglioma.

Treatment

Treatment for a low-grade oligodendroglioma is similar to that for a low-grade astrocytoma. Ideally, all or almost all of the tumor should be surgically removed.

After surgery, you'll be reevaluated for your next treatment (called adjuvant treatment). Your next type of treatment will be based on the risk of the tumor to regrow:

- **Low risk** – A person who is under 40 years old and whose tumor has been removed completely is considered to have a lower risk for the tumor to regrow. Someone with a low-risk tumor could enter a clinical trial or be under observation after surgery.
- **High risk** – A person who is over age 40 or has had a partial resection is at higher risk. The best adjuvant treatment option may be a clinical trial. Otherwise, the next treatment is usually radiation

therapy followed by chemotherapy (PCV or temozolomide). Another option is radiation and chemotherapy given at the same time.

Follow-up

After treatment, you'll have regular MRI or CT scans to make sure the tumor hasn't grown. The usual schedule for follow-up scans is every 3 to 6 months for a few years, and then every 6 months if the tumor remains stable. The scans will also monitor the health of your brain and identify any side effects of radiation therapy or chemotherapy.

Recurrence

The signs and symptoms of your oligodendroglioma may disappear for months or even several years after treatment. However, most grade 2 oligodendrogliomas eventually evolve into high-grade oligodendrogliomas over time. For more about the recurrence of low-grade oligodendrogliomas, *see Chapter 6*.

Other low-grade gliomas

Other low-grade gliomas include pilocytic astrocytoma, pleomorphic xanthoastrocytoma, subependymal giant cell astrocytoma, ganglioglioma, and more. These gliomas are rare in adults and not covered in this book.

"My doctor encouraged me to seek additional medical opinions to ensure I was comfortable with my treatment decision."

Key points

- Seizure is the most common symptom of low-grade gliomas. However, many people with low-grade gliomas have no symptoms.
- The main treatment for a low-grade glioma is surgery to remove all of the tumor or as much of it as possible.
- Grade 2 glioma tumors don't have clearly defined edges. This makes them difficult to remove entirely by surgery.
- Oligodendrogliomas are diagnosed by the combination of two biomarkers: *IDH* mutation and 1p/19q co-deletion.
- Although low-grade gliomas grow slowly, many eventually become high-grade gliomas.

5

Treatment for high-grade glioma

A high-grade glioma can come on quickly and grow rapidly. People with a high-grade glioma often have a poor prognosis. However, many people with these tumors are now living longer than the statistics suggest.

About high-grade gliomas

Most gliomas that occur in adults are high grade. High-grade gliomas are malignant (cancerous), rapidly growing grade 3 or grade 4 tumors. Grade 3 gliomas include astrocytomas and oligodendrogliomas. Grade 4 gliomas include astrocytomas and glioblastomas. These are aggressive, life-threatening gliomas.

Symptoms of grade 3 and grade 4 tumors can come on quickly. Symptoms may be due to the tumor as well as the swelling around the tumor pressing on the brain. This can cause nausea, vomiting, and severe headaches that are worse in the morning or in the middle of the night.

The location of the tumor can also affect symptoms. For instance, a high-grade tumor located near the motor cortex of the frontal lobe can affect movement or cause weakness on one side of the body. Seizures are another common symptom of these gliomas.

If the results of your MRI show what looks like a high-grade glioma, you should be able to meet with a multidisciplinary team that will work with you to come up with a treatment plan.

Developing a treatment plan may involve further examination and testing before therapy can begin. An essential part of testing is obtaining a biopsy of the glioma to confirm the type of tumor. Surgically removing most of the tumor (resection) may also be an option at this point.

Tumor surgery

The main goal of a resection is to relieve pressure on the brain and safely remove as much of the tumor as possible. This is called maximal safe resection. Your treatment team will look closely at your MRI scan to decide whether maximal safe resection is possible for you. Your team will also consider other factors to determine the safety of this operation. These factors may include your performance status, your age, how fast the tumor is growing, and more.

The two possible types of tumor surgery are:

- **Maximal safe resection** – The goal of this surgery is to safely remove as much of the tumor as possible. This may involve awake surgery during which the neurosurgeon will stimulate critical areas of the brain near the tumor. Within a day or two after the surgery, you'll have another MRI scan to find out how much of the tumor was removed.
- **Partial resection or biopsy** – If your treatment team thinks maximal resection isn't possible or isn't a good option

for you, then you might have a partial resection or a biopsy (stereotactic biopsy or open biopsy). Within a day or two after the partial resection, you'll have another MRI scan to find out how much of the tumor remains.

In either type of resection, the neuropathologist will examine the tissue sample from your tumor. Histologic and biomarker tests will indicate what type of glioma you have.

Types of high-grade glioma tumors include oligodendrogliomas, astrocytomas, and glioblastomas.

High-grade oligodendroglioma

High-grade oligodendrogliomas are typically rapidly growing, grade 3 gliomas. High-grade oligodendrogliomas often have a better prognosis than other high-grade gliomas.

Oligodendrogliomas may appear almost anywhere in the central nervous system but often develop in the frontal or temporal lobes of the brain.

Biomarkers

Molecular testing can reveal specific biomarkers that may enhance the diagnosis, prognosis, and treatment of a high-grade oligodendroglioma. Notably, the combination of an *IDH* mutation and a 1p/19q co-deletion is necessary to diagnose an oligodendroglioma.

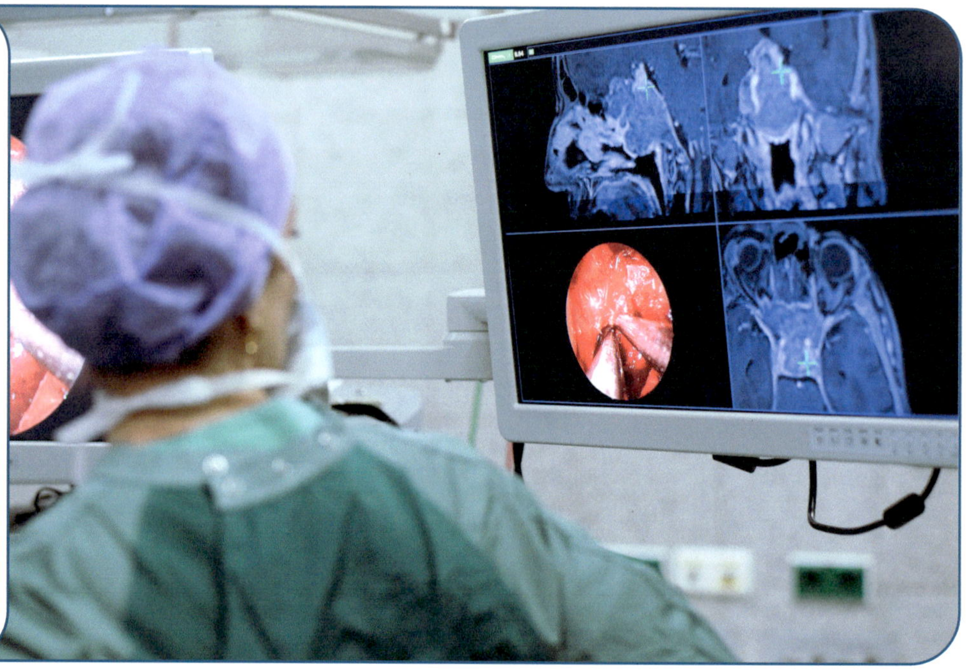

Imaging aids surgery

To precisely guide surgery, a computer programmed with imaging scans can pinpoint the exact location of a brain tumor.

- ***IDH*** – An *IDH* mutation in a grade 3 oligodendroglioma indicates a better chance for longer survival.
- **1p/19q** – Chemotherapy is likely to work better in a glioma that has a 1p/19q co-deletion.
- ***TERT* promoter** – A *TERT* promoter mutation, when it occurs along with *IDH* mutation and 1p/19q co-deletion, helps confirm the diagnosis of oligodendroglioma.
- ***MGMT* promoter methylation** – In high-grade gliomas, temozolomide chemotherapy generally works better in tumor cells with a methylated *MGMT* promoter than in those with an unmethylated *MGMT* promoter.

Treatment

Surgery to try to remove the tumor is the first step of treatment. Because a high-grade oligodendroglioma blends into the surrounding brain tissue, removing the entire tumor usually isn't possible. So you'll have additional treatment (called adjuvant treatment) to destroy as many of the remaining tumor cells as possible.

You can consider joining a clinical trial to receive additional treatment. If a clinical trial isn't an option, then the adjuvant treatment for a high-grade oligodendroglioma is usually radiation plus chemotherapy.

Your treatment team may recommend one of these options:

- Radiation therapy either before or after PCV (procarbazine, lomustine, and vincristine) chemotherapy
- Radiation therapy followed by temozolomide chemotherapy
- Radiation therapy and temozolomide chemotherapy given together, followed by more temozolomide chemotherapy

People who are older or who have limited physical capability (low performance status) may not be able to handle both radiation and chemotherapy. One of these less intense adjuvant treatments may be a better option:

- Radiation therapy (possibly concentrated into a shorter period of time) with or without temozolomide chemotherapy
- Temozolomide chemotherapy only
- Supportive (palliative) care

Follow-up

After treatment, you'll need to have regular MRI scans to find out if the oligodendroglioma is under control. These scans can also monitor the health of your brain and identify any side effects of radiation or chemotherapy. Scans are scheduled every 2 to 4 months for a few years, and then every 3 to 6 months if there's no recurrence.

Recurrence

A high-grade oligodendroglioma is likely to come back eventually. When it does, it may be even more aggressive. For more about recurrence, *see Chapter 6*.

High-grade astrocytoma

High-grade (grade 3 and grade 4) astrocytomas are rapidly growing gliomas. The cells in these tumors have changed so much that they no longer look like normal glial cells.

In addition, grade 4 astrocytomas often have necrosis, which is an area of dead tumor tissue. Grade 4 astrocytomas can also grow a large amount of new blood vessels, which feed their fast growth. Finding either or both of these features suggests the astrocytoma is more severe and is growing faster than a grade 3 astrocytoma.

High-grade astrocytomas occur in almost any part of the central nervous system. But they're most often located in the brain's frontal or temporal lobes.

Biomarkers

Specific biomarkers of high-grade astrocytomas include:

- ***IDH*** – An *IDH* mutation in a high-grade astrocytoma generally indicates longer survival and a better outcome from radiation therapy or chemotherapy.
- ***ATRX*** – An *ATRX* mutation that occurs with an *IDH* mutation can help confirm the diagnosis of astrocytoma.
- ***MGMT* promoter methylation** – In high-grade astrocytomas, temozolomide chemotherapy generally works better in tumor cells with a methylated *MGMT* promoter than in those with an unmethylated *MGMT* promoter.
- ***CDKN2A/B*** – Deletion of *CDKN2A* and *CDKN2B* genes is a trait that helps diagnose grade 4 astrocytomas. This is important to know because a grade 4 astrocytoma grows more quickly and has a more serious prognosis than lower-grade astrocytomas.

Treatment

Surgery to try to remove the tumor (either maximal or partial resection) is the first step of treatment for a high-grade astrocytoma.

Because high-grade astrocytomas invade the surrounding brain tissue, removing the entire tumor won't be possible. So additional (also called adjuvant) treatment is needed. The purpose of additional treatment is to destroy as many of the remaining tumor cells as possible.

Your additional treatment could be receiving therapy in a clinical trial. NCCN experts recommend that anyone with a high-grade glioma consider a clinical trial for adjuvant treatment. If a clinical trial isn't available or possible, then additional treatment usually means radiation plus chemotherapy.

Depending on your situation, your treatment team may recommend one of these options:

- Radiation therapy followed by temozolomide chemotherapy
- Radiation therapy and temozolomide chemotherapy given together, followed by more temozolomide chemotherapy
- Radiation therapy and temozolomide chemotherapy given together, followed by more temozolomide chemotherapy plus alternating electric field therapy (grade 4 astrocytoma only)
- Radiation therapy alone (grade 4 astrocytoma only)

People who are older or who have limited physical capability (low performance status) might benefit from less intense therapy instead. Less intense treatment options include radiation therapy only (possibly concentrated into a shorter period of time), temozolomide chemotherapy only (which is preferred for people who have the *MGMT* promoter methylation biomarker), or simply supportive care.

Follow-up

After treatment, you'll need to have regular MRI scans to find out if the astrocytoma is under control. These scans also monitor the health of your brain and identify any side effects of treatment. Scans are scheduled every 2 to 4 months for a few years, and then every 3 to 6 months if there's no recurrence.

Recurrence

Although treatment may stop or slow the tumor for a while, a high-grade astrocytoma is likely to come back. Or it may continue to grow despite treatment. For more information about recurrence, *see Chapter 6.*

What is the blood-brain barrier?

Your brain is a very important organ. It needs special protection to keep it safe and healthy. To block germs, infections, and other toxins from getting in, the brain has a unique security system. This protective layer is called the blood-brain barrier. It's like a moat that surrounds and protects a castle.

The blood-brain barrier does its job well—maybe too well. One problem with the barrier is that it won't permit most drugs in the blood to reach the brain. This includes many chemotherapy drugs. However, scientists have learned that some chemotherapy drugs can cross the blood-brain barrier more easily than others. Some of these drugs are used to treat gliomas.

Even so, doctors and scientists are constantly investigating new and better ways to send drugs through the blood-brain barrier to reach brain tumors.

Glioblastoma

Glioblastomas are fast-growing and aggressive grade 4 tumors. They're the most common and the most dangerous type of malignant brain tumor in adults.

Glioblastomas don't usually evolve from lower-grade gliomas—they typically emerge as grade 4 tumors right from the beginning (de novo). Glioblastomas can occur anywhere in the brain or spinal cord, but they develop most often in the temporal and frontal lobes of the brain.

Glioblastomas are highly infiltrative—they expand and merge deep into the surrounding brain tissue.

Glioblastomas are characterized by areas of dead cells (necrosis). They also produce a large amount of new blood vessels to feed their fast growth. Because glioblastomas grow quickly, they need to be diagnosed and treated as soon as possible.

Biomarkers

A glioblastoma has one or more of these biomarkers:

- ***IDH*** – One clue to identifying a glioblastoma is that it **doesn't have** an *IDH* mutation.
- ***TERT* promoter** – Most glioblastomas have a mutation in the *TERT* promoter. Finding this biomarker helps predict the prognosis of the disease.
- **7 gain/10 loss** – The combination of gaining chromosome 7 and losing chromosome 10 is a strong identifying biomarker of glioblastoma.
- ***MGMT* promoter methylation** – Nearly half of glioblastomas have *MGMT* promoter methylation. Finding this biomarker is important for treatment. A glioblastoma with a methylated *MGMT* promoter tends to respond better to temozolomide chemotherapy and leads to longer survival compared with a glioblastoma with an unmethylated *MGMT* promoter.
- ***EGFR*** – Mutations in the *EGFR* gene occur frequently in glioblastoma, which makes this a helpful biomarker for diagnosis.

Treatment

As with other gliomas, the first treatment for glioblastoma is to try to surgically remove most of the tumor. But because glioblastoma cells invade so deeply into brain tissue, removing the entire tumor won't be possible. So additional treatments are needed. In some individuals, carmustine wafers could be inserted after the tumor tissue is surgically removed.

The purpose of additional treatment (also called adjuvant treatment) is to destroy as many of the remaining tumor cells as possible. NCCN experts highly recommend that people with glioblastoma consider a clinical trial as part of their treatment plan. If a clinical trial isn't possible or available, additional treatment usually involves radiation, chemotherapy, and other therapies.

Adjuvant treatment for older adults (over age 70) is often different than treatment for adults under age 70. In general, older adults are given less intense treatment. There are several reasons for this. Many older adults have additional health problems, limited physical capability (lower performance status), reduced mental functioning, or a greater risk of developing side effects.

Keep in mind that people over age 70 aren't all the same and aren't all treated the same. Some adults over age 70 can tolerate more intense treatment and get good results. No matter what your age or condition is, your treatment team will help you determine the best type of additional treatment for you.

Here are the most common adjuvant treatment options for glioblastoma based on age and physical ability:

Under age 70, with good physical capability – People under age 70 who have good performance status are generally able to handle stronger adjuvant treatment. Options include joining a clinical trial or having one of these treatments:

- Radiation therapy and temozolomide chemotherapy given together, followed by more temozolomide chemotherapy plus tumor treating fields (TTFields)
- Radiation therapy and temozolomide chemotherapy given together, followed by more temozolomide chemotherapy
- Radiation therapy and lomustine/temozolomide chemotherapy given together, followed by more lomustine/temozolomide chemotherapy
- Radiation therapy only

Under age 70, with limited physical capability – People under age 70 who have lower performance status are generally given less intense adjuvant treatment. You can see if you can join a clinical trial. Or you can have one of these treatment options:

- Hypofractionated (larger doses in fewer sessions) radiation therapy with or without temozolomide chemotherapy given at the same time or afterward
- Temozolomide chemotherapy only
- Supportive (palliative) care

Over age 70, with good physical capability – People over age 70 who have good performance status are generally given a modified level of treatment. Options include joining a clinical trial or having one of these treatments:

- Hypofractionated radiation therapy and temozolomide chemotherapy given together, followed by more temozolomide chemotherapy
- Standard radiation therapy and temozolomide chemotherapy given together, followed by temozolomide chemotherapy plus TTFields
- Temozolomide chemotherapy only
- Hypofractionated radiation therapy only

Over age 70, with limited physical capability – People over age 70 who have lower performance status are generally given less aggressive treatment that minimizes side effects. In addition to a clinical trial, adjuvant treatment options may include:

- Hypofractionated radiation therapy only
- Temozolomide chemotherapy only
- Supportive care

Follow-up

After treatment, you'll need to have regular MRI scans to find out if the glioblastoma is under control. These scans also monitor the health of your brain and identify any side effects of radiation or chemotherapy. Scans are scheduled every 2 to 4 months at first, and then 3 to 6 times a year if there's no recurrence.

Recurrence

Eventually, the glioblastoma will likely come back. Or it may continue to grow despite treatment. For more information about recurrence, *see Chapter 6*.

"Keeping a journal is a low-cost and practical tool to help you navigate this frightening and uncertain time. By tracking your daily symptoms, you are in a better position to see how you're doing over time, which can be clouded by one or two bad days."

Quality of life

Quality of life refers to a person's overall enjoyment of life, including their sense of well-being and ability to participate in their usual activities.

Your quality of life should be the main priority that guides your treatment and care. Successful treatment isn't just about reducing the cancer. Other goals include minimizing cognitive problems, reducing pain, lowering anxiety and stress, carrying out regular activities, being with friends and family, and enjoying life as best as you can.

Key points

- High-grade gliomas are rapidly growing and possibly life-threatening tumors.
- The main goal of high-grade glioma surgery is to relieve pressure on the brain and safely remove as much of the tumor as possible.
- Surgically removing all of a high-grade glioma won't be possible because these tumors have grown deep into the surrounding brain tissue.
- NCCN experts recommend that anyone with a high-grade glioma consider a clinical trial as part of their treatment plan.
- A high-grade oligodendroglioma is identified by the combination of two biomarkers: *IDH* mutation and 1p/19q co-deletion.
- Glioblastomas are the most common and the most dangerous of the gliomas. More than half of all gliomas in adults are glioblastomas.
- In general, older and/or frail adults receive less aggressive treatment. But there are exceptions to this—every person's case is different.

6
Recurrence and progression

For most people who've been treated for a glioma, the tumor will come back even after treatment (recurrence). Or the tumor may keep growing despite treatment (progression). Here's how you and your treatment team can manage recurrence or progression.

After the intense activity and frequent appointments involved with treatment, you'll begin a new phase of recovery: "watching and waiting." This quieter, less busy time can also be stressful in its own way. Shifting from the active process of treatment to the inactive period of waiting and wondering can be difficult.

No one knows if, when, or how your tumor may come back. So it's important to keep going to follow-up appointments. You'll have periodic imaging scans as well as regular physical and neurological exams.

For most people, gliomas eventually do return. Very often, the glioma comes back with greater intensity and faster growth than before.

Low-grade glioma

If you have a low-grade glioma (grade 1 or grade 2) that continues to grow or comes back after treatment, you'll require additional treatment aimed at minimizing the tumor. Your multidisciplinary care team will meet again and discuss the best options for you.

Depending on your situation and what therapy you've had before, a recurrent or progressive low-grade glioma can be treated with one or more of these options:

- Clinical trial
- Surgical resection or biopsy
- Radiation therapy plus chemotherapy
- Chemotherapy only
- Radiation therapy only
- Observation (for low-risk disease)
- Supportive care

High-grade glioma

If you have a low-grade glioma that comes back as a high-grade glioma (grade 3 or grade 4) or if you have a high-grade glioma that progresses or comes back, there are still options to treat the tumor. Surgical resection may be possible for certain tumors, such as large tumors or those located all in one area (local tumor).

Otherwise, treatment options for recurrent or progressive high-grade glioma include:

- Clinical trial
- Chemotherapy
- Radiation therapy plus chemotherapy
- Targeted therapy
- TTFields (for glioblastoma only)
- Supportive care

In certain individuals, more radiation therapy might be an option. Another option in certain cases is chemotherapy combined with targeted therapy.

Rehabilitation

Because gliomas can impair areas of the brain that control important senses and skills—like speech, vision, hearing, movement, and thinking—you may need rehabilitation after treatment. These health professionals can provide:

Physical therapy – Involves training to improve movement, balance, and walking, and increase strength.

Occupational therapy – Will assist you in regaining your ability to do day-to-day activities, such as working or taking care of household tasks.

Speech therapy – Can help you with difficulties in your ability to speak and communicate.

Low vision therapy – For problems such as vision loss, double vision, and blind spots.

Neuropsychiatric care – Helps with changes in mood, behavior, thinking, problem-solving, memory, and more.

What is pseudoprogression?

Pseudoprogression occurs when imaging scans show that the tumor appears to be growing after treatment, but what looks like tumor growth on the images is actually a reaction to treatment.

It can be difficult for your doctors to tell the difference between pseudoprogression and real tumor progression based on imaging alone. This is a common situation, and it can be very stressful. Additional imaging or having another biopsy or surgery may be necessary to confirm whether the tumor is truly progressing.

What's next?

You could have several types of treatment for a relapsed or progressive glioma. After any treatment, it's important to go to follow-up visits and stay in touch with your treatment team.

You may eventually reach a point where you want to stop treatment. For some people, how they spend their time is more important than how much time they have left.

It's common to feel frustration, anger, regret, despair, and uncertainty—even all at the same time. Know that you can have a brain tumor and still find happiness after diagnosis and treatment. Try to enjoy life as much as possible. Talk with family or friends. Join a support group to learn how other patients are dealing with their cancer. Or talk to your doctor or another member of your care team. They can point you to professionals who can help you deal with these feelings and guide you toward your next steps.

> **"It's easy to lose your sense of identity when you have a brain tumor. Find something that 'feels like you'—reading, yoga, being with family, whatever—and get back to that thing as quickly as you can. Recovering a sense of self amidst the uncertainty of a brain tumor diagnosis can help us maintain our resilience in the face of challenges."**

Supportive care is appropriate for anyone, regardless of age, cancer stage, or the need for other therapies. For more information about supportive care and other resources, turn to the next chapter.

Because gliomas can impair areas of the brain that control important senses and skills—like speech, vision, hearing, movement, and thinking—you may need rehabilitation after treatment.

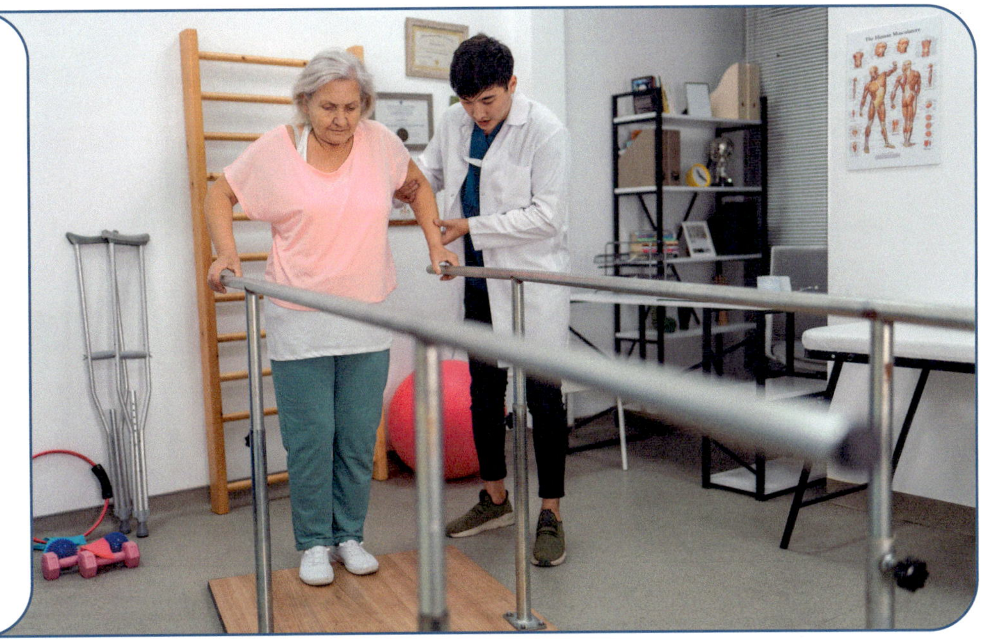

Key points

- Follow-up involves periodic imaging scans as well as regular physical and neurological exams.
- For most people, gliomas eventually do return. Very often, the glioma comes back with greater intensity and faster growth than before.
- Recurrence is when a tumor comes back after effective treatment.
- Progression is when the tumor keeps growing despite treatment.
- It's common for people with cancer to feel frustration, anger, regret, despair, and uncertainty—even all at the same time.
- Supportive care is appropriate for anyone, regardless of age, cancer stage, or the need for other therapies.

"Please allow yourself to accept hard days, difficult moments, or disappointments. Speaking with a behavioral health specialist can help you to prepare for the emotional changes that you may face."

7 Supportive care

Supportive care addresses the symptoms and side effects of cancer and cancer treatments, as well as psychological, social, financial, and spiritual issues. Many resources are available to help you feel better and answer your questions.

The main concern for most patients with cancer is to find a treatment that works. Having cancer is about more than just treatment, though. Cancer care can be a rollercoaster that includes many additional physical and emotional challenges. It's important to know that you can get support for these challenges.

What is supportive care?

Supportive care (also called palliative care) is for controlling cancer symptoms, relieving the suffering that comes with the diagnosis and treatment of cancer, and improving the quality of life for those with cancer and their loved ones and/or caregivers.

Supportive care is given at any stage of disease, not just at the end of life.

Supportive care involves the whole person, not just their cancer. Supportive care addresses many needs. Notably, supportive care can help prevent or treat physical and emotional symptoms. It can assist with making treatment decisions and coordinating care between health providers. It can provide aid for psychological, social, and spiritual issues. Supportive care can help you find support groups or patient advocacy organizations. It also helps with finding assistance for financial support, legal issues, advance care planning, and end-of-life concerns.

Ask questions and reach out to your treatment team if you need more information about supportive care. Some medical centers have patient navigators or other staff members who coordinate nonclinical supportive care.

Anxiety and depression

Depression, anxiety, fear, and distress are very common feelings for people with gliomas—as well as their loved ones and caregivers. You may feel anxious or experience depression during a hard part of treatment or because your life is different than it was before your brain tumor. These feelings can make it harder to deal with a brain tumor and with tumor treatment. They can hold you back even when you want to move forward.

Tell your treatment team if you're experiencing these symptoms. Getting help when you're feeling worried or hopeless is an important part of your care. Help can include support groups, talk therapy, or medication. Patient navigators, social workers, and other experts at your medical center can help. Some people also feel better by exercising, talking with loved ones, or relaxing.

Read more about cancer and distress in *NCCN Guidelines for Patients: Distress During Cancer Care*, available at NCCN.org/patientguidelines and on the NCCN Patient Guides for Cancer app.

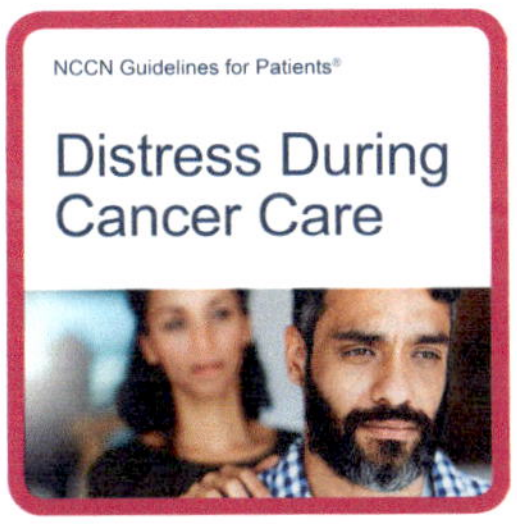

Support groups

Many people diagnosed with a brain tumor find support groups to be helpful. A support group provides the opportunity to talk with others who are going through, or have been through, similar experiences. Support groups often include people at different stages of treatment. Some people may be newly diagnosed, while others may be finished with treatment.

In a support group, people with common ground share information on their experiences, financial and emotional burdens, coping strategies, and knowledge about research and treatments. A support group can also be a good source of practical advice and helpful tips.

Ask your doctors or supportive care team about finding a brain tumor support community. If your hospital or community doesn't have support groups for people with brain tumors, have a look at the online resources listed on *page 65* of this book.

"Do whatever you can to connect with a support group. Being diagnosed with a brain tumor can be scary. It is priceless to be able to discuss diagnosis, treatment, or living with a tumor with someone who has gone through similar experiences as you have."

Financial concerns

The financial cost of a brain tumor can be overwhelming. As a result, many people with brain tumors and their loved ones struggle with the cost of treatment, as well as the stress of paying for it.

If you struggle to pay for food, housing, treatment, follow-up care, and other expenses, or you have difficulty getting to appointments, talk with your care team's social worker, patient navigator, and hospital financial services staff. Many patient advocacy groups also have resources. They can help you find financial support and transportation options.

You can also talk to your treatment team about time off from work, health insurance, or money problems. Your team can include information in your treatment plan to help you manage your finances and medical costs. If your doctors and care providers don't talk about how to pay for treatment, it's OK for you to ask them about it first.

Survivorship

Survivorship focuses on the health and well-being of a person with a brain tumor, from diagnosis until the end of life. This includes the physical, mental, emotional, social, and financial effects of the brain tumor that begin at diagnosis, continue through treatment, and arise afterward.

Survivorship also includes concerns about follow-up care, late effects of treatment, tumor recurrence, and quality of life. Support from family members, friends, and caregivers is also an important part of survivorship.

Read more about survivorship in *NCCN Guidelines for Patients: Survivorship Care for Healthy Living* and *Survivorship Care for Cancer-Related Late and Long-Term Effects*, available at NCCN.org/patientguidelines and on the NCCN Patient Guides for Cancer app.

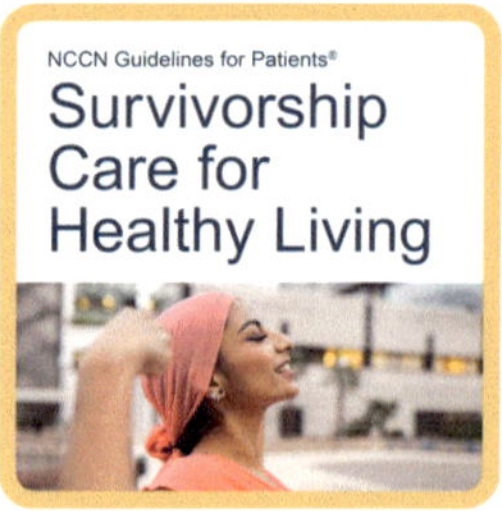

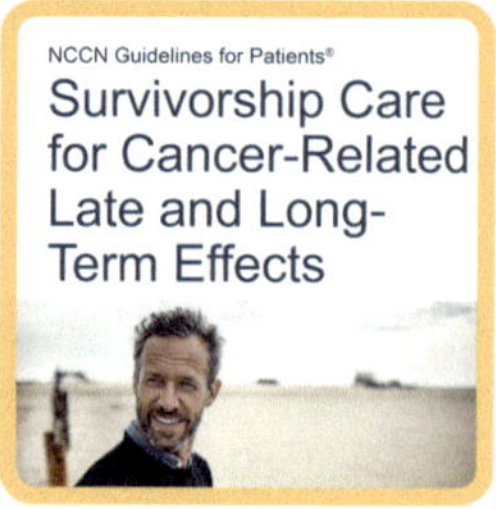

“Report any unusual feelings of sadness, loss of interest in activities, anxiety, and sleep problems to your doctor. Many people experience these feelings, and they should not go untreated.”

Advance care planning

When a glioma is diagnosed at an advanced stage or keeps progressing despite all treatment efforts, it may be time to consider what lies ahead. Even when brain tumors are curable, talking about future scenarios should begin when starting treatment. This exploration of what’s important to you is called advance care planning.

Advance care planning is for everyone, not just for those who are very sick. Advance care planning means deciding what care you would want if you become unable to make medical decisions for yourself. It’s about making sure that your wishes are understood and respected. Patients with brain tumors can set up an advance care plan early to help them feel less stressed and better able to cope with their condition.

End-of-life considerations

End-of-life care provides medical, psychological, and spiritual support for people who are close to the end of life as well as the people who love them. The goal is comfort, not a cure. It may also be called comfort care or hospice.

Note that hospice is a special kind of end-of-life care. Hospice refers specifically to an insurance benefit for people whose life expectancy is 6 months or less. Hospice supports those at the end of life by bringing in additional care providers and resources such as home care.

Providing support for family members is a key part of hospice care. Most programs offer counseling and support groups for family members, including support after the patient has died. It can be very comforting to know that your loved ones will have that kind of support after you're gone.

For more information about **supportive care**, **advance care planning**, and **end-of-life concerns**, see *NCCN Guidelines for Patients: Palliative Care*, available at NCCN.org/patientguidelines and on the NCCN Patient Guides for Cancer app.

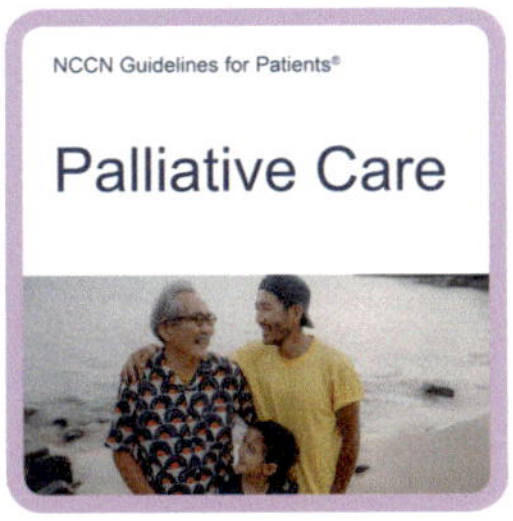

"Don't be afraid to accept help from friends and family."

Key points

- Supportive care is for relieving symptoms and side effects, and for other health issues related to brain tumors.
- Supportive care is given at any stage of disease, not just at the end of life.
- Supportive care is treatment that involves the whole person, not just their brain tumor.
- For help with financial support and transportation options, talk with your care team's social worker, patient navigator, and hospital financial services staff.
- Survivorship focuses on the health and well-being of a person with a brain tumor from diagnosis until the end of life.
- Advance care planning is done to ensure that your end-of-life wishes are understood and respected.
- Hospice care is for people who are close to the end of life. It's focused on comfort and quality of life.

8

Making treatment decisions

It's important to be comfortable with the treatment you choose. This choice starts with having an open and honest conversation with your care team.

It's your choice

Treatment decisions are very personal. What is important to you may not be important to someone else.

In shared decision-making, you and your care team share information, discuss the options, and agree on a treatment plan. It starts with an open and honest conversation between you and your team.

Some things that may play a role in your decision-making:

- What you want and how that might differ from what others want
- Your religious and spiritual beliefs
- Your feelings about certain treatments like surgery or chemotherapy
- Your feelings about pain or side effects
- Cost of treatment, travel to treatment centers, and time away from school or work
- Quality of life and length of life
- How active you are and the activities that are important to you

Think about what you want from treatment. Discuss openly the risks and benefits of specific treatments and procedures. Weigh options and share concerns with your care team. If you can build a relationship with your care team, you'll feel supported when considering options and making treatment decisions.

Second opinion

It's normal to want to start treatment as soon as possible. While treatment for a glioma shouldn't be postponed or ignored, there is usually enough time to have another care provider review your test results and suggest a treatment plan. This is called getting a second opinion. It's a normal part of health care. Even doctors get second opinions!

Things you can do to prepare for a second opinion:

- Check with your insurance company about its rules on second opinions. There may be out-of-pocket costs to see doctors who are not part of your insurance plan.
- Make plans to have copies of all your records sent to the provider or specialist you will see for your second opinion.

Questions to ask

Possible questions to ask your care team are listed on the following pages. Feel free to use these or come up with your own. Be clear about your goals for treatment and find out what to expect from treatment.

Questions about cancer testing

1. What tests will I have?
2. Do the tests have any risks?
3. Will my insurance pay for all of the tests you're recommending?
4. What should I do to prepare for testing?
5. Should I bring someone with me to the appointments?
6. Where do I go for testing, and how long will it take?
7. If any of the tests will hurt, what will you do to make me comfortable?
8. Do you offer genetic testing for tumors? If not, where do you refer patients for genetic testing of their tumor?
9. How soon will I know the results and who will explain them to me?
10. How can I get a copy of the pathology report or access my results online?

Questions about treatment options

1. What are my treatment options?
2. Does any option offer a cure or long-term cancer control?
3. Is a clinical trial an option for me?
4. Are you suggesting options other than what NCCN recommends? If yes, why?
5. How do my age, sex, overall health, and other factors affect my options?
6. What will happen if I do nothing?
7. What if I am pregnant, or planning to become pregnant?
8. What can be done to prevent or relieve the side effects of the treatments?
9. How do I get a second opinion?
10. How long do I have to decide about treatment, and is there a social worker or someone who can help me decide?

Questions about resources and support

1. Who can I talk to about help with housing, food, and other basic needs?
2. What assistance is available for transportation, childcare, and home care?
3. Who can tell me what my options for health insurance are and assist me with applying for insurance coverage?
4. How much will I have to pay for my treatment? What help is available to pay for medicines and other treatments?
5. Who can help me with my concerns about work or school?
6. How can I connect with others and build a support system?
7. Who can I talk to if I don't feel safe at home, at work, or in my neighborhood?

Questions about what to expect

1. Does this hospital or cancer center offer the best treatment for me?
2. Do I have a choice of when to begin treatment?
3. How long will treatment last?
4. Will my insurance cover the treatment you're recommending?
5. Are there any programs to help pay for treatment?
6. What supportive care and services are available to me and my caregivers?
7. Who should I contact with questions or concerns if the office is closed?
8. How will you know if my treatment is working?
9. What are the chances of my glioma worsening or returning?
10. What follow-up care is needed after treatment?

Questions about side effects

1. What are the possible complications and side effects of treatment?
2. Which side effects are most common and how long do they usually last?
3. Which side effects are serious or life-threatening?
4. Are there any long-term or permanent side effects?
5. What symptoms should I report right away, and who do I contact?
6. What can be done to prevent or relieve the side effects of treatment?
7. Do any medications worsen side effects?
8. Do any side effects lessen or worsen in severity over time?
9. Will you stop or change treatment if there are serious side effects?

Questions about clinical trials

1. How do I find clinical trials that I can participate in?
2. What are the treatments used in the clinical trial?
3. Has the treatment been used for other types of cancer?
4. What are the risks and benefits of this treatment?
5. What side effects should I expect and how will they be managed?
6. How long will I be in the clinical trial?
7. Will I be able to get other treatment if this doesn't work?
8. How will you know if the treatment is working?
9. Will the clinical trial cost me anything?

Questions about your care team's experience

1. Are you board certified? If yes, in what area?
2. What is your experience as well as your team's experience with treating the type of cancer I have?
3. How many patients like me (of the same age, gender, race) have you treated?
4. Will you be consulting with experts to discuss my care? Who will you consult?
5. Is this treatment (or procedure) a major part of your practice? How often have you done this treatment (or procedure) in the last year?
6. How many of your patients have had complications? What were the complications?

Resources

CancerCare
Cancercare.org

Cancer Hope Network
Cancerhopenetwork.org

MedlinePlus
medlineplus.gov/cancers.html

National Cancer Institute
cancer.gov

National Coalition for Cancer Survivorship
canceradvocacy.org

Triage Cancer
Triagecancer.org

Words to know

adjuvant therapy
Additional treatment given after the main treatment to lower the chances of the cancer returning.

advance care planning
Making decisions now about the care you would want to receive if you become unable to make medical decisions or to speak for yourself.

alternating electric field therapy
A treatment that uses low-intensity energy to stop tumor cells from multiplying. Also called tumor treating fields (TTFields).

astrocytoma
A glioma that looks like small, star-shaped cells (astrocytes) found in the central nervous system.

biomarker
Any chemical, substance, or other sign in your body that can be measured to assess your health.

biopsy
A procedure that removes fluid or tissue samples to be tested for a disease.

central nervous system
The brain and spinal cord.

chemotherapy
A drug treatment that damages and destroys rapidly dividing cells throughout the body.

chromosomes
The structures within cells that contain coded instructions for cell behavior.

clinical trial
A research study that assesses how well health tests or treatments work in people.

computed tomography (CT)
An imaging test that uses x-rays from many angles to make a picture of the inside of the body.

diagnosis
The identification of an illness based on tests.

follow-up care
Health care that involves regular check-ups, which begin after treatment has ended.

glioblastoma
A fast-growing, malignant, high-grade tumor found in the central nervous system.

glioma
A malignant tumor that develops from brain cells called glial cells.

high-grade glioma
A rapidly growing grade 3 or grade 4 brain tumor that develops from glial cells.

imaging
A technology that makes pictures (images) of the insides of the body.

infusion
A method of giving drugs slowly through a needle into a vein.

low-grade glioma
A slower-growing grade 1 or grade 2 brain tumor that develops from glial cells.

magnetic resonance imaging (MRI)
An imaging process that uses a magnetic field and radio waves to make pictures of the inside of the body.

multidisciplinary care
A treatment method where doctors, specialists, and other health providers work and communicate as a team to provide expert care for the patient.

mutation
An abnormal change in the genetic code (DNA) of a gene within cells.

neuropathologist
A doctor who specializes in testing cells and tissue of the central nervous system to find disease.

observation
A period of testing for changes in cancer status while not receiving treatment.

oligodendrocytes
Glial cells that cover and protect nerve cells in the brain and spinal cord.

oligodendroglioma
A slower-growing glioma that looks similar to oligodendrocytes in the central nervous system.

performance status
A rating of a person's overall health and ability to do ordinary activities.

prognosis
The likely course and outcome of a disease.

progression
The growth or spread of cancer after being treated.

pseudoprogression
The appearance on imaging that a tumor is growing when it's actually shrinking after treatment.

radiation therapy
A treatment that uses intense energy to destroy tumor cells.

recurrence
The return of disease after a period of improvement.

refractory cancer
Cancer that does not improve with treatment.

relapse
The return of cancer after a period of improvement.

remission
The absence of cancer signs and symptoms after treatment.

resection
Surgical removal of tissue.

supportive care
Health care for the symptoms of cancer and the side effects of cancer treatment. Also called palliative care.

surgical (resection) margin
The normal tissue around the edge of a tumor that is removed during surgery.

targeted therapy
A drug treatment that identifies and attacks a specific feature of cancer cells.

tumor
A mass of abnormal cells.

tumor grade
A rating based on how different tumor cells look from normal cells under a microscope. It's used to predict how fast the tumor is likely to grow.

NCCN Contributors

This patient guide is based on the NCCN Clinical Practice Guidelines in Oncology (NCCN Guidelines®) for Central Nervous System Cancers Version 1.2023. It was adapted, reviewed, and published with help from the following people:

Dorothy A. Shead, MS
Senior Director
Patient Information Operations

John Murphy
Medical Writer

Laura Phillips
Graphic Artist

The NCCN Clinical Practice Guidelines in Oncology (NCCN Guidelines®) for Central Nervous System Cancers Version 1.2023 were developed by the following NCCN Panel Members:

Louis Burt Nabors, MD/Chair
O'Neal Comprehensive Cancer Center at UAB

Jana Portnow, MD/Vice-Chair
City of Hope National Medical Center

Joachim Baehring, MD
Yale Cancer Center/Smilow Cancer Hospital

Ankush Bhatia, MD
University of Wisconsin Carbone Cancer Center

Orin Bloch, MD
UC Davis Comprehensive Cancer Center

Steven Brem, MD
Abramson Cancer Center at the University of Pennsylvania

Nicholas Butowski, MD
UCSF Helen Diller Family Comprehensive Cancer Center

Donald M. Cannon, MD
Huntsman Cancer Institute at the University of Utah

Samuel Chao, MD
Case Comprehensive Cancer Center/ University Hospitals Seidman Cancer Center and Cleveland Clinic Taussig Cancer Institute

Milan G. Chheda, MD
Siteman Cancer Center at Barnes-Jewish Hospital and Washington University School of Medicine

Andrew J. Fabiano, MD
Roswell Park Comprehensive Cancer Center

Peter Forsyth, MD
Moffitt Cancer Center

Pierre Gigilio, MD
The Ohio State University Comprehensive Cancer Center - James Cancer Hospital and Solove Research Institute

Jona Hattangadi-Gluth, MD
UC San Diego Moores Cancer Center

Matthias Holdhoff, MD, PhD
The Sidney Kimmel Comprehensive Cancer Center at Johns Hopkins

*Craig Horbinski, MD, PhD
Robert H. Lurie Comprehensive Cancer Center of Northwestern University

Thomas Kaley, MD
Memorial Sloan Kettering Cancer Center

*Michelle Kim, MD
University of Michigan Rogel Cancer Center

Ryan Merrell, MD
Vanderbilt-Ingram Cancer Center

Maciej M. Mrugala, MD, PhD, MPH
Mayo Clinic Comprehensive Cancer Center

Seema Nagpal, MD
Stanford Cancer Institute

Lucien A. Nedzi, MD
St. Jude Children's Research Hospital/ The University of Tennessee Health Science Center

Kathryn Nevel, MD
Indiana University Melvin and Bren Simon Comprehensive Cancer Center

Phioanh L. Nghiemphu, MD
UCLA Jonsson Comprehensive Cancer Center

*Ian Parney, MD, PhD
Mayo Clinic Comprehensive Cancer Center

*Toral R. Patel, MD
UT Southwestern Simmons Comprehensive Cancer Center

Katherine Peters, MD, PhD
Duke Cancer Institute

Vinay K. Puduvalli, MD
The University of Texas MD Anderson Cancer Center

Chad Rusthoven, MD
University of Colorado Cancer Center

*Nicole Shonka, MD
Fred and Pamela Buffet Cancer Center

Lode J. Swinnen, MBChB
The Sidney Kimmel Comprehensive Cancer Center at Johns Hopkins

Stephanie Weiss, MD
Fox Chase Cancer Center

Patrick Yung Wen, MD
Dana-Farber Cancer Institute

*Nicole E. Willmarth, PhD
American Brain Tumor Association

NCCN

Mary Anne Bergman
Guidelines Coordinator

Susan Darlow, PhD
Manager, Guidelines Information Standardization

Senem Kurtoglu Lubin, PhD, MBA
Oncology Scientist/Medical Writer

* Reviewed this patient guide. For disclosures, visit NCCN.org/disclosures.

NCCN Cancer Centers

Abramson Cancer Center
at the University of Pennsylvania
Philadelphia, Pennsylvania
800.789.7366 • pennmedicine.org/cancer

Case Comprehensive Cancer Center/
University Hospitals Seidman Cancer Center and
Cleveland Clinic Taussig Cancer Institute
Cleveland, Ohio
UH Seidman Cancer Center
800.641.2422 • uhhospitals.org/services/cancer-services
CC Taussig Cancer Institute
866.223.8100 • my.clevelandclinic.org/departments/cancer
Case CCC
216.844.8797 • case.edu/cancer

City of Hope National Medical Center
Duarte, California
800.826.4673 • cityofhope.org

Dana-Farber/Brigham and Women's Cancer Center |
Mass General Cancer Center
Boston, Massachusetts
617.732.5500 • youhaveus.org
617.726.5130 • massgeneral.org/cancer-center

Duke Cancer Institute
Durham, North Carolina
888.275.3853 • dukecancerinstitute.org

Fox Chase Cancer Center
Philadelphia, Pennsylvania
888.369.2427 • foxchase.org

Fred & Pamela Buffett Cancer Center
Omaha, Nebraska
402.559.5600 • unmc.edu/cancercenter

Fred Hutchinson Cancer Center
Seattle, Washington
206.667.5000 • fredhutch.org

Huntsman Cancer Institute at the University of Utah
Salt Lake City, Utah
800.824.2073 • healthcare.utah.edu/huntsmancancerinstitute

Indiana University Melvin and Bren Simon
Comprehensive Cancer Center
Indianapolis, Indiana
888.600.4822 • www.cancer.iu.edu

Mayo Clinic Comprehensive Cancer Center
Phoenix/Scottsdale, Arizona
Jacksonville, Florida
Rochester, Minnesota
480.301.8000 • Arizona
904.953.0853 • Florida
507.538.3270 • Minnesota
mayoclinic.org/cancercenter

Memorial Sloan Kettering Cancer Center
New York, New York
800.525.2225 • mskcc.org

Moffitt Cancer Center
Tampa, Florida
888.663.3488 • moffitt.org

O'Neal Comprehensive Cancer Center at UAB
Birmingham, Alabama
800.822.0933 • uab.edu/onealcancercenter

Robert H. Lurie Comprehensive Cancer Center
of Northwestern University
Chicago, Illinois
866.587.4322 • cancer.northwestern.edu

Roswell Park Comprehensive Cancer Center
Buffalo, New York
877.275.7724 • roswellpark.org

Siteman Cancer Center at Barnes-Jewish Hospital
and Washington University School of Medicine
St. Louis, Missouri
800.600.3606 • siteman.wustl.edu

St. Jude Children's Research Hospital/
The University of Tennessee Health Science Center
Memphis, Tennessee
866.278.5833 • stjude.org
901.448.5500 • uthsc.edu

Stanford Cancer Institute
Stanford, California
877.668.7535 • cancer.stanford.edu

The Ohio State University Comprehensive Cancer Center -
James Cancer Hospital and Solove Research Institute
Columbus, Ohio
800.293.5066 • cancer.osu.edu

The Sidney Kimmel Comprehensive
Cancer Center at Johns Hopkins
Baltimore, Maryland
410.955.8964
www.hopkinskimmelcancercenter.org

The UChicago Medicine Comprehensive Cancer Center
Chicago, Illinois
773.702.1000 • uchicagomedicine.org/cancer

The University of Texas MD Anderson Cancer Center
Houston, Texas
844.269.5922 • mdanderson.org

UC Davis Comprehensive Cancer Center
Sacramento, California
916.734.5959 • 800.770.9261
health.ucdavis.edu/cancer

UC San Diego Moores Cancer Center
La Jolla, California
858.822.6100 • cancer.ucsd.edu

UCLA Jonsson Comprehensive Cancer Center
Los Angeles, California
310.825.5268 • uclahealth.org/cancer

UCSF Helen Diller Family
Comprehensive Cancer Center
San Francisco, California
800.689.8273 • cancer.ucsf.edu

University of Colorado Cancer Center
Aurora, Colorado
720.848.0300 • coloradocancercenter.org

University of Michigan Rogel Cancer Center
Ann Arbor, Michigan
800.865.1125 • rogelcancercenter.org

University of Wisconsin Carbone Cancer Center
Madison, Wisconsin
608.265.1700 • uwhealth.org/cancer

UT Southwestern Simmons
Comprehensive Cancer Center
Dallas, Texas
214.648.3111 • utsouthwestern.edu/simmons

Vanderbilt-Ingram Cancer Center
Nashville, Tennessee
877.936.8422 • vicc.org

Yale Cancer Center/Smilow Cancer Hospital
New Haven, Connecticut
855.4.SMILOW • yalecancercenter.org

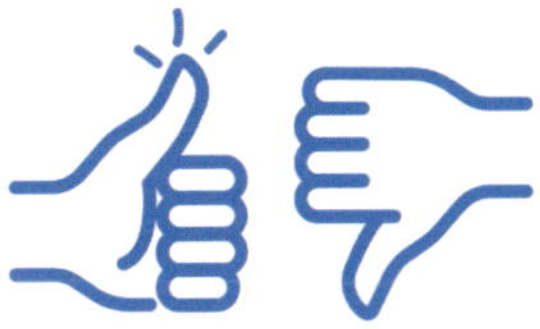

Let us know what you think!

Please take a moment to complete an online survey about the NCCN Guidelines for Patients.

NCCN.org/patients/response

Index

Made in the USA
Monee, IL
03 June 2026

51648316R00045